Find Your P

MW00413801

For Estheticians and Massage Therapists

By Grace J Power

Acknowledgments:

Thank you Sean Stenson for supporting me in completing my first book and helping take care of Stellar so I had some quiet time to write. I love you.

Thank you Kathryn Reynolds for editing my book and encouraging me with the content.

Thank you Rachelle Jasmine for everything you do for the company so I have more free time to focus on writing.

Thank you Ben Fuchs for being so generous in formulating creams for me, and your encouragement to help other estheticians in business.

Thank you Seven Grey for designing the front cover of my book and your help promoting it online.

Thank you Fyll Callan for helping me expand My Gold Sugar to more estheticians and for your friendship.

Thank you T Harv Eker for creating and leading my first Millionaire Mind Intensive and teaching me how to increase my money blueprint.

Chapters:

Introduction:

If you picked up this book, it probably means you are a massage therapist or esthetician looking to increase your financial success. We often get into the business because we want to help people, but we find out we can't give away our services for free, at least not all the time. We do need to find a way to create an income to support our business expenses as well as our life.

Whether you are just starting out or already have a full schedule of clients, this book will help you discover the importance of a niche. Having a niche not only increases your profitability, but most of the time gives you more energy because you are working with your favorite clients, and doing your favorite services. It helps give you clarity and focus in how to brand and market your business. *Having a niche will set you apart and make it easier for you to be successful in the industry.* Through reading this book you will be inspired in how to determine your unique niche and be exposed to the bigger vision of what's possible for your short term and long term future as a successful esthetician or massage therapist.

About the Author:
Grace J Power is a massage therapist and esthetician. She started into the industry in 2002 and made over $50,000 her first year as a massage therapist starting her business from scratch at the age of 21. She then went on to attain her esthetician license and bought a Day Spa business. That is where she discovered her niche of doing Brazilians. Shortly after, she sold the Day Spa and founded Acomoclitic Hair Removal Studio. In eight years, Grace sold the hair removal studio after hitting over a half million in annual sales. She is now 34 and a full time mom with a two year old son. She has three product lines that she promotes online, producing sales all over the USA and into other countries around the world. Having been successful, Grace finds fulfillment in helping other massage therapists and estheticians find their niche and prosper. Keep reading to discover some of the secrets to her wealth and how you can follow in her footsteps with your unique expertise.

Chapter 1: Choosing Your Niche

Oftentimes your niche will come to you naturally. Other times, you may need to go out and find it. For me it was a combination. I had heard from T Harv Eker, author of Secrets to the Millionaire Mind, that having a niche will actually bring you more profit in business. *You may feel as though you are limiting your possibilities, but you are actually increasing them by picking a niche.* I decided to trust this guidance.

At the time I owned a day spa where we offered a full menu of services. Being new to the industry, I kept adding more services every few months. I was so excited about everything, I wanted to try it all. When I initially bought the spa they offered facials, waxing, massage and nails. From there I added body wraps, spray tanning, acupuncture, permanent make up, hot stone massage, Brazilian waxing for women and men, and I was in the process of adding laser hair removal and photofacials when I sold it. By adding so many things, it made it difficult to brand which made it difficult to market.

While working at the spa, I was the only esthetician who wanted to do Brazilians. All the other estheticians were intimidated or not interested in offering them. I began to notice that my Brazilian clients were really fun! I was able to talk to them the whole time and oftentimes they would share with me personal things about their life. This never happened when I did massages and facials. I usually was quiet the majority of the time for those services. But Brazilian waxing was unique. Because it was rather painful during parts, the clients also grew a stronger trust in me. They knew the service would hurt, but they were trusting that I would get the job done without causing more pain or discomfort than necessary. Through this process, I created a bond with my Brazilian clients that was much deeper than my massage clients.

I noticed the financial benefits to offering Brazilians especially as I picked up speed and could do a Brazilian in 30 minutes or less. I was charging the same amount of money for a Brazilian as I was for an hour long massage or facial. Plus, Brazilian clients would come back month after month as their hair would grow back in. If they went longer than a month, the process was more painful so there was incentive to not miss a month.

After hearing T Harv Eker's advice about having a niche, I started thinking about opening a studio that specialized in doing Brazilians. I started researching immediately. Then I started putting together a business plan. I met with a few other business owners and shared my ideas with them. Having their ideas as well helped me solidify my plans. Next thing I knew I was registering my new business name for Acomoclitic Studio and putting a deposit down on a space for rent. Everything was coming together.

As I built my business from the ground up, I noticed that it was very easy and fun to do the branding and marketing since I had such a narrow niche of male and female Brazilians. I was offering laser hair removal and waxing in the beginning (eventually sugaring replaced waxing). Besides Brazilians, I did hair removal on all the areas of the body, but the majority of my clients came in for Brazilians and then added on other areas if needed. I was having so much fun because instead of doing all sorts of various services throughout the day, I was only doing hair removal and I was gaining expertise and efficiency.

I'm so happy and I've been so successful, I want to share it with you. I want to see other estheticians, massage therapists, and people in our industry excel in their businesses. *With all the variety of services, products and target markets, everyone can have a unique niche and be successful at it.*

In our industry, your niche could be a specific service, a specific target market, or a specific product. Some examples are:

Massage Therapy and Skin Care for Professional Golfers
Massage Therapy for Pre and Post Pregnancy
Massage Therapy for Elderly
Energy work for Anxiety and Depression
Esthetician who specializes in Permanent Eyeliner
Esthetician who specializes in Electrology for Hormonal Hair
Problems
Esthetician who specializes in Skin Cancer care, treatments and
prevention
Esthetician who specializes in Adult Acne

The more specific you can be, the more success you will have in
branding and marketing yourself.

When choosing a niche to focus in on, you will want to consider these six questions:
1. What are you passionate about?
You want to choose something that ignites you. For me it was
Brazilians. I loved the relationships I could make with the
customers and I loved the feeling of being trusted with such an
intimate service. It could be that your niche is something you are
already doing but you want to be doing more of. Or perhaps it's
something you see is missing in the marketplace...something you
have heard is in demand but no one has specialized in it yet. Even
though it may not be something you are really passionate about at
the moment, after looking into it further, you may discover it is your
golden ticket and it has you smiling just thinking about it.
Passion is important because you are going to be spending
countless hours formulating, creating, selling and being involved in
your business. You want it to be something you are going to love
every single day.
I never get tired of selling Brazilians. I want everyone (especially
the women) to try it out. I know how great they are and I love
offering them to people. I also love selling My Pink Wink Cream
and Sugaring. I am passionate about these products. They make
me so happy. I have caught myself kissing the bottles

occasionally. That is how much I love them!

When I first started doing Brazilians, I used hard wax and I thought it was the best. My passion for offering Brazilians grew to a whole new level once I started sugaring. Both my clients and I benefited from a much more efficient, less painful and cleaner process. I was in heaven....and so were my clients.

If you aren't sure what you are passionate about, take some time to notice what services you get the most excited about when you see them on the schedule. *Another way to start determining your passion, is to notice what services you are **not** excited about.* If you get super excited about doing hydro-facials but you don't like doing regular facials, that is a clue. If you notice that you feel sick working on acne skin but you really enjoy when clients add on a skin tightening mask, that is a clue.

Even though I enjoyed facials and massage, I was so much more excited about waxing, in particular Brazilian waxing. That is how I knew it was a passion and something that I would enjoy doing as my niche. If you are brand new to the industry, you may not have had a chance to experience all the varieties of services, products or clients, so you may want to work at a spa first to try some different things out before you focus in on your niche business. More than likely though, you started to get a feel for what you enjoyed the most and what things you didn't really like doing as much when you were going through school or working in the field. That is a great starting point.

You will notice that you have a lot more energy when you create a business where the majority of your day you get to do what makes you the most excited, you will do a better job at the service and your clients will pick up on your excitement and passion and be much more likely to rebook and refer people to you. *You may have heard the saying "follow your bliss"; that is what I would recommend when choosing your niche business.*

2. What are the start up costs?

Even though passion is important, you also want your niche to make business sense. Start up costs include anything you need to purchase or invest in to get into business. You want to consider all the costs because even the little things can really start to add up. Some ideas include: registering your business, trademarking your business name, logo design, business card design and printing, brochure design and printing, website design, rent plus deposit, remodeling a space, lighting, equipment, instruments, back bar supplies, sheets, products, retail items, office supplies, phone, internet, laptop, software, printer, filing system, furniture, decor, reception area, product shelving, etc.

Obviously, you don't need every little thing before you take on your first client. What I did, and teach others to do, is to start small and use the money that comes in to add and upgrade things as you go. I did this with Acomoclitic from day one and it's fun to look back at the pictures of when I first opened with barely anything. Over the years I transformed the space to be more functional and attractive. I worked with five different designers, two different lighting companies, an architect, sign companies, electricians and handymen. I kept improving the space little by little every year, as to not spend too much money all at once. Every time I spent money on the space, I asked myself, do I want to spend this money on my business or towards a personal expense? One time I had the choice of adding in sinks in the treatment rooms and decided to use that money instead towards a ten day trip to Australia and New Zealand. It turned out that I never once missed having the sinks in the rooms, and scuba diving in the barrier reef was an experience I will never regret. If you don't pace yourself, it's easy to spend $30,000 all in one go in remodeling, signage, and decorating costs. Instead, spread this out over years to avoid going broke your first year in business. I always kept my vision of what I truly wanted, but didn't rush getting there. Eventually I reached my goals and by not starting with everything all at once, it gave my clients something to look forward to. Clients like seeing a business that keeps current and has something new each time they visit. It's a sign of progress and success. Even if it is simply rearranging your products and highlighting different products and services.

The best thing to do to calculate your start up costs, is to write down the 'absolutely necessary' costs, the 'need it fairly quickly' costs, the 'eventually I will need it' costs and the 'someday I would like it' costs. By doing this, you will not be so intimidated by the total start up costs because you will be able to see how it can be gradually purchased instead of all up front.

If you are not sure of the costs for some of the things you want for your business, you can start by writing down an anticipated cost range. Then go back later and do some research to get more specific. Looking for things like used equipment instead of new equipment could be an option to start at lower initial costs. You can always upgrade as you grow your business. There are companies that will lease equipment so that you don't have to come up with the full price to get started. I did this with my lasers and LAM probe machine at Acomoclitic.

When I started my first massage business, I didn't have much money saved - basically enough for my first month's rent. My massage table was included in my massage school tuition. The only other start-up cost was purchasing sheets and massage oil. I started out with the bare minimum. The only decor I had was a picture on the wall that I brought from home. I remember my room having a very flat, "echoey" sound because of the tile floors and the only furniture I had was a chair and a massage table. As the money came in from the customers, I used that money to add some decor. It was a super small room though, so I couldn't fit too much.

In our industry, you really can get started with the bare minimum. Even if you start with doing massage at your house or your client's house, all you really need is the massage table, sheets and some oil. If you are doing facials, you can start with what you are using on your own skin. When I first introduced facials, I took my facial cleanser and toner from my bathroom to use on my first clients. I offered a deal with doing a facial and a massage in one hour. While the steam was going I did the arm and shoulder massage. While the mask was sitting on, I did the leg massage. So needless to say, don't let the start up costs keep you from launching your niche business. It's wise to expect some start up costs so you aren't blindsided, but, in our industry, you can pretty much get started with what you have. If needed, you could even give massages or facials, on the floor or on a bed in the beginning. If you treat it like a business from the beginning, you will make money and you will grow a loyal clientele that will follow you as you move into bigger and better accommodations for them. *Even if you start less professional than what you would like, keep the vision and it will come to fruition.*

On a final note, even though I never earned a loan or grant, I did apply for them. It never hurts to try and see if you can qualify for a grant which you don't have to pay back, or a low interest loan, like an SBA loan. But don't count on this money to get started. And some of the loans are a long process to apply for, so while you are waiting, start offering your services.

3. What are the per service costs?

When choosing your niche, your cost for the services that are going to be your specialty should be profitable. You want your revenue to be able to cover all your costs and pay you a nice income. Take into account the time and product costs for delivering the service, along with what equipment is required. Make sure that when all is accounted for, you are making a profit. One of my friends has a business in which she primarily does microdermabrasion and uses the LAM probe machine that treats any minor skin irregularity. She has clients on a set program where the first visit they receive the microdermabrasion and the full face spot treatment. Then a follow up microdermabrasion is scheduled a couple weeks later. The skin is reassessed and she recommends when the next spot treatment needs to be done. She has her own product line that she sells her clients to improve the results from the services they receive. Her entire business revolves around two machines that are not very expensive and deliver amazing results!

By having a niche, you may be able to charge more (i.e. Aveda Salons) because it is your specialty, or you may be able to charge less (i.e. Massage Envy) because you have such a streamlined system that beats out the competition. Every niche service is going to be different. However, carefully considering the per service costs will help you set your prices accurately including your promotional, membership or package pricing. If you do have employees, whether receptionists or technicians, you will need to account for all of those costs as well.

If, for some reason, you have a great niche idea, but at the end of all the calculations it doesn't look like a profitable one, brainstorm with some other people; either come up with a way to cut costs, increase prices, or discover a different niche entirely. Sometimes the craziest niches that seem impossible to be profitable can actually become incredibly profitable with the right timing, marketing, persistence, or plain luck. Don't be too quick to throw away a great niche idea just because the numbers don't quite compute. Oftentimes, the entrepreneur's spirit of "where there's a will, there's a way," might have you find a twist that makes you successful with it.

If you plan on eventually hiring staff to do the services for you as your business grows, you will want to consider the costs of paying them. Additionally, when I hired estheticians to do the Brazilians, the tip income was not really 'income' anymore since that money went to the esthetician. You will want your prices set so that you still profit after you pay the employee their wages and the tips. Prices can always be adjusted down the road, but it still is something to consider, especially if you are offering memberships or package pricing that could affect your profit when hiring staff later on.

4. Who is your target market?
Another important factor to consider are the clients. What clients do you enjoy working with the most? Who are the clients that really make your day? You could have a whole business based around your target market. If you are drawn to work with golfers, you could have multiple services and products offered that appeal to that demographic. For instance, imagine a little spa that

specializes in care for golfers. It would be strategically located near or at a golf club offering products and services that address sun exposure and the common injuries golfers experience; such as facial services that would help alleviate a sunburn; body treatments that could address sun exposure on legs or the back of the neck; massage treatments that focused on the common areas where golfers experience soreness; and hot/cold treatments or ultrasound treatments that could address injuries. Sun block would be a great seller. By selling or giving away products with your logo on them such as hats, sunglasses or even golf shirts and shorts, the clients would become a walking billboard for you while on the golf course.

Can you see how easy it would be to put together your marketing materials knowing you wanted to target golfers? It would also be so much easier to know where to advertise and what other businesses you could affiliate with who share the same target market. The website content would be easier to create. Each blog article could be about a specific health and wellness concern for golfers and promote a product or service that offers a solution for that concern.

Even the descriptions of the services on your brochure or website could describe how the service was addressing a golfer. The names of some of your products could be creative with golf terms such as *The Green* Facial Mask or *Hole in One* Hand Cream.

I'm not sure about you, but I find it to be so much fun coming up with all sorts of new ideas. If it overwhelms you, you can always start with the very basics and add more variety as you grow your clientele. *In fact, the clients are oftentimes the best resource for your new ideas.*

As you can imagine, if all of your marketing was aimed at golfers and you offered a superior service customized to their needs, why would they not go to you?

Choosing your target market will also set the tone for your business. If you go after women in politics versus pursuing engineers, you are going to have different types of conversations with your clientele and a different tone altogether in the environment that will appeal to them. Before you go after a certain group just because you think they will have the money to afford your services, make sure they are the type of person you really enjoy serving.

In my personal experience, I enjoyed my Brazilian clients so much more than my facial and massage clients. When I owned Acomoclitic, we did a photofacial promotion on Groupon and so we had a lot of new clients coming in for photofacials. At the next staff meeting, we all agreed that we didn't enjoy these new clients as much as we enjoyed new clients who came in for Brazilians. So from then on, I didn't promote photofacials to new clients. I only promoted them to our existing clients.

When I was sculpting my target market, I was clear about what type of people I wanted to work with based on the kinds of Brazilian clients I was seeing at the spa. I wanted to work with people who were fun, open minded, sexual, loving, self aware, positive and beautiful. From there I discovered that these types of people tended to be in sales, in business, in a steady career, or working as a waitress or in the beauty industry.

You can gather some ideas of who your target market is from the people you know are currently getting the services that you want to create your niche in. Another example of using your target market as your niche is brides. You could provide specific services tailored to brides, bridal parties, bachelorette parties, and the family of the bride. Or you could narrow down your niche even more to something like 'The Groomed Groom' and offer hair, skin, nail, and hair removal services for grooms preparing for their big day and honeymoon. This opens up your affiliate opportunities to every business who targets the bride and weddings. Just from these examples, you can see how much fun it is to have a niche and how much easier marketing becomes when you know specifically who your target market is and what specific services you provide for them.

oftentimes as you narrow down your target market, you actually find more facets to it that other companies aren't harnessing. As you work more with your target market, you will discover more about what they like and want from you. If their suggestions excite you and offer you additional revenue, you can incorporate them into your business because they are still within your niche. When putting together your business plan, you will want to specify your target market and as your business grows, keep referring back to your original plan. It's easy to get distracted and off course. With every new marketing material or print ad, ask yourself, "Am I attracting my target market with this?" You will notice yourself choosing specific advertising avenues because they already are targeting your niche market. This will increase the response you have on your advertising. Plus the business you do pull in will be more likely to become repeat customers and refer people to you because you met their specific need, and were the best at it.

5. Who is your competition?
Competition is not a bad thing. The narrower your niche, the more you see other professionals in your industry as your comrades instead of your competition. In fact, I've never really liked that word because oftentimes there are ways to work with the so called 'competition' and turn them into comrades. One example of this is when I was completely booked and had clients that couldn't wait until my next opening, I was able to send them to my competition who I trusted instead of saying, "There isn't anything that I can do for you." Clients are often surprised by the referral, but also grateful since they may have a hard time finding a trusted place simply looking online or in a directory.

I've also had an occasional potential client who asked for a referral closer to where they lived and I gave them the name of a salon or esthetician who I trusted. When a client moves to another city, they have sometimes asked me who they should go to. It's pretty easy to go online and find someone near them who offers a similar service with either the same equipment, products or techniques that I use, so I will do this for them since they may not know exactly what to search for. In return, I have had multiple estheticians and two Denver waxing salons send their customers to Acomoclitic Studio for similar reasons.

Another example of how we teamed up with our competition is when we had an inappropriate male client and we immediately asked him to leave. He had mentioned going to another salon during the consultation, so I called them and asked if they had made note of a similar experience with this client. They said they hadn't, but that he had just called trying to get in. Fortunately, they didn't have any openings that day. She made a note on his account in case he were to call again in the future. I'm sure they appreciated the warning!

I read one time about a hair salon who had a great policy for problem clients. If they had a client who they couldn't please, they would give them a gift certificate to a neighboring salon. I thought this was a great idea! I haven't done that exactly, but I did have a tough customer who wanted really cheap laser prices and complained about how far we were from her. I went online and found a couple places closer to her home that used our same laser and recommended them to her. This may seem like a bad business decision, but I didn't regret it. Sometimes it's simply not worth the hassle of trying to accommodate someone that another business is better suited for.

Massage therapists can work with each other by sending clients back and forth who may be a better fit for the others' style. If you like doing Deep Tissue, it is helpful to have a trusted massage therapist that you can send clients who want Swedish to. It's also helpful if you share a room and have different styles. That way by sending each other occasional clients, you still help yourself by ensuring the other portion of rent is paid, and they are more likely to refer clients back to you.

When putting together your business plan, you will want to research your competition. And even after getting your business started, you will want to constantly keep up on what other companies are doing in your industry and especially your niche. Remember that any services you get from other salons and spas while spying on what they are doing, is a tax deduction. I include it as "Market Research." It is actually rather fun to investigate your competition to gather new ideas for what you want to do the same or differently. For instance, I have heard over and over again that other wax salons do not get all the hair and they don't get out ingrowns. These are two things that I incorporated into Acomoclitic. We pride ourselves in getting all the hair (including the butt crack hair on Brazilians). We also schedule extra time to allow time for removal of any ingrown hairs, and do a thorough check to make sure we didn't miss anything. Quite a few of the wax salons in the Denver area only schedule 15 minutes for a Brazilian. We normally schedule 30-45 minutes. Another simple thing that I would hear about other estheticians who waxed, was that they didn't put their hand down on the skin immediately after pulling out the hair. This is one thing that we are able to incorporate and make the experience much less painful for our customers. It seems so simple and yet it makes a difference for them and many clients have told us that it is one of the reasons they come back to us and don't want to go anywhere else.

Your competition is not only those businesses that are located near you physically, but also those businesses that come up on search engines for specific keywords. Brainstorm strategies for how you will compete with these other companies. When you have a niche, that is one way that you will eliminate much of your competition. You want to be the only one that has your exact specialty. I eliminated much of my competition with other spas and salons by narrowing down to Brazilian hair removal, sugaring, anal bleaching and Vadazzeling. I also haven't heard of any places around that offer the Cheek Glow which is basically a facial for the butt cheeks. These simple things set us apart online so we stood out above our competition for our unique specialities. To stand out online for your niche, it would be helpful to have the 'word' people would search for in your title. When I first opened, my business name was Acomoclitic Laser & Wax Studio (before I started offering sugaring), so it was easier for people to recognize the services I offered from the name. If I was just called Acomoclitic Studio, it would have been harder for my website and Google listing to rank high when people searched for Laser or Wax Services. Also, if people saw the listing Acomoclitic Studio, they wouldn't have known for sure what services we did and perhaps would not have called or clicked to get more information. By having Laser and Wax in the name, it helped me pop up higher on Google searches for those search terms and also made it clear to the customer what services I offered. Especially in the beginning, when you are growing your business and wanting to be recognized for a specialty, it really helps to have the name of the service in your business name. You could always change the name down the road once you have established clientele, if desired. For example, let's say you want to be known for massage for the elderly, you wouldn't want to call your business "Comfort Touch" because that isn't quite clear and doesn't help with online searches for massage or for senior citizens. In the beginning, it would be more advantageous to have a name like "Golden Age Massage for Seniors."

When choosing a niche, especially if it is very specific, you may find that you have no competition, at least for that particular niche. When I started offering Sugaring at Acomoclitic, we were one of the only places in the Denver area that offered sugaring. Now there are more places that offer it, but it is still much harder to find than waxing. One thing I noticed was that people new to the area who had been sugared in their previous home town, sought out sugaring in Denver and would drive quite a distance sometimes, past all of the waxing salons because they only wanted to be sugared. I also had male clients driving quite a distance because we were one of the only places around that really promoted men's Brazilians on our website.

Knowing who your competition is will help you determine your pricing. I would often look and see what other places charged for the same services that I was offering. Since so many people can shop online now, that is a great place to start your search. There are many people in our industry that don't have a web presence yet, and perhaps don't need one if they are already completely booked up. If they are in the same niche as you, seek them out so that you can find out their prices and anything else they are doing that is working well for them in filling their schedule. Depending on your situation, you may want to price higher or lower than the competition. Oftentimes, people who specialize in a specific service can charge higher prices because they are the expert and clients will pay more for their knowledge and experience. If this is the route you choose to go, keep in mind that you can always do special promotions and discounts in the beginning to attract new clients, but as long as your customers know these are promotional prices, they won't be shocked or angry when you charge them your high price on future visits.

In other cases, you may want to charge lower prices for your niche service because you are so efficient, but then charge higher prices for the services you don't want to promote. For instance, when I first started my Brazilian hair removal studio, I would charge $95 for an hour massage which was on the high end because I didn't want to attract massage clients. In fact, I didn't even have massage as a service listed on my menu, but I did have clients ask about it since I was a massage therapist. So in the beginning, before I was booked solid with hair removal services, I would give massages to those clients who asked and were willing to pay $95 per hour. I noticed that I didn't mind doing the massage when I felt like I was being compensated well for it. Once I was accustomed to making $55 in 15 minutes for a wax or $100 for a 5 minute laser, I didn't want to go back to doing an entire hour of massage for only $60 which was the average rate.

Charging a lower rate than average for your niche services can make them more affordable to accommodate a broader range of income levels. By having more competitive pricing, it also opens up more opportunity for repeat business when they are priced so the average person can afford them on a monthly basis. For instance, if you were able to do a perfect brow shaping in 8 minutes or less, you could book 8 people in an hour and charge ten bucks each and still make $80 plus tips per hour. Plus, the majority of those people would be re-booking with you every 2-4 weeks at that price. Once you were booked solid for as many hours as you wanted to work, you could either raise your prices slightly, or train someone else in your methods and help them get booked up and if you paid them $20 per hour plus their tips, you would still be making $60 per hour without working harder. When you can keep your prices competitive and it is a service you are highly skilled and trained in, it's a recipe for success.

When it came to pricing, I can't know for sure if I 'did it right.' When the Groupon craze started, it really changed the laser hair removal industry and I ended up slashing my advertised prices on my menu and website to compete. Looking back, I wonder if I would have been better off keeping the higher prices and doing Groupon-type specials? That way the customer would see the value they were getting. I could have kept the higher price listed with a slash through it and then the special price in red next to it. That being said, it's always helpful to stay aware of the competition and strategize how you are going to compete. You don't want to find that you are spinning your wheels trying to get your business going, only to find out it's not working because of your advertised pricing. Let's say you want to charge $100 for your service. When you look at the competition, they are only charging $50, but you know they aren't including everything into it that you do, and they aren't as skilled as you. One thing you could do to compete, is to charge $50 on your menu, but then charge additional pricing for the 'upgrades' that you want to include. Once you have the client in your treatment room and you have established the relationship with them with you as the expert, it will be easier for you to explain the benefits of the upgrades and sell them to the client. If you don't have anyone in your treatment room because your prices are too high, then try out this strategy to help fill your schedule.

In my case of doing Brazilian waxing, I noticed that some other salons would charge additional fees for trimming the hair, removing ingrowns, applying an ingrown hair solution, or if the service took more time because the person was extra hairy, or adding the abdomen trail or doing the full bikini line (which might include inner thighs). My strategy was to include all of those extras in my regular service and win repeat business because they received an exceptional experience at the same price they would pay somewhere else that didn't include all the 'upgrades'. The only thing I did charge extra for was when I had to do the entire buttcheek area, but I would always ask the customer first and let them know I charged an additional $20 for that area so they could choose. That strategy worked and it fit with my personality. I would not have been able to let a client leave without getting out their ingrown hairs. I also could not wax someone without trimming the hair first. I'm sure some salons don't give the clients a choice in the matter and just charge them the extra fees when they check them out. If the client is caught off guard by the higher price, they may feel like they were taken advantage of and not return.

Setting prices could be the determination of success or failure, so it is a very important part of setting up your business and studying your competition to see what they are doing, especially the businesses that are most successful.

6. Where will you be located?

We have all heard it said "location, location, location" and oftentimes location can make or break a business. Your online 'location' can be even more important than your physical location, especially as a small business. However both are important and something that you will want to put some attention towards.

My first business was doing massages. I was in a women's fitness center. My treatment room was smack dab in the middle of all the commotion; chatty ladies locker room on one wall, aerobic classroom on another, and the nursery on the other wall. It was not the ideal place for a quiet, relaxing massage room. In spite of all that I was able to have a steady client base and repeat business. My first year in business in 2002, I brought in just over $50,000 in revenue building my business from scratch. Some of the positives to this location were being located in an affluent area, having a built-in client potential with the members at the gym, and the gym was in a strip mall right off a busy highway. I asked the gym if I could offer massages for non-members and we worked out a win-win situation. I charged a non-member rate so there was incentive for them to become members. This allowed me to advertise in a local magazine; that is one way I brought in quite a bit of new business. Since I couldn't do male clients at the women's gym, I worked out a deal with a chiropractor in the same shopping center that I could use his facility for massages on a commission basis. I started gaining some regular clients that were covered by insurance at his office. It was a little more work because I had to bring over my massage table and my supplies to set up for the massages, but at least it was conveniently located. My second year in business, I ended up working with another chiropractor closer to my house. He was just starting a brand new business and did all the advertising for me. He was located in a busy shopping center and also did mass print advertising. He paid me on commission plus tips. I split my time between both the women's gym and his office. I set up an interesting schedule where I flip-flopped mornings and evenings at both places, so essentially I would end up doing 6-8 massages per day with a break in the middle to have lunch and drive to the other location. I noticed that by reducing my hours at the women's gym, my schedule was almost always booked solid. And because the chiropractor was doing so much promotion for me, I was booked up at his office as well. When I decided to go to esthetician school, I hired two massage therapists, one for each location to take over my day appointments and help on weekends. Hiring massage therapists was fun because I had a handful of free massages before I decided on the top two candidates, both of them were awesome...actually even better than me as far as their knowledge and understanding of the human body. The therapist I hired for the chiropractic office did more Deep Tissue massage than I did. She couldn't have been able to do 8 massages per day, but she could handle 3-4 which was all I needed her for since I covered the evening clients. The therapist I hired for the women's fitness center had a very similar touch as I did, even though she was half my height. I'm over six feet tall and she was about four feet tall. While going to esthetician school, I was still able to do 3-4 massages every evening alternating between both offices and then full days on Saturday and Sunday. When I started working on the floor at esthetician school, I couldn't keep working Saturdays, so the other therapists helped out more.

I say all of this, partly to share my story, but also to point out that having multiple locations can help expand your customer reach. I was located in high traffic areas that were easy to get to and see from major highways and intersections. I think that played an important part in my success. Especially since the internet was not as prominent then as it is today. My brother actually built a website for me with some great pictures of my office and me doing massages, but it wasn't high ranking online and it really didn't bring in a ton of traffic. It was used more as a brochure to make my business cards more useful by having the link listed if people were interested to check out more before calling to schedule. However the location didn't seem to do the women's gym much good. Within a month after I moved out, I drove by and found the building empty. They had gone out of business. Obviously, it takes more than location to make a business successful. I think in their case, the overhead was too much. I was only paying $400 per month for a small room and their rent was closer to $3,000 per month so they had to sell a lot of memberships to just pay rent!

I have found online location is becoming even more important than brick and mortar location. Your online location includes things like your website address, your blog, your social media page, Youtube channel, Google maps listing, Yelp page, and of course your organic search placement for specific keywords relating to your business and your niche. Like most people starting a new business, you might not have a lot of extra funds to invest in building a website. Even though it's something you will want to have, you could easily get started with free things like a Facebook page, a blog and a Youtube channel. All of those things don't cost anything to start, and it's a great way to list your phone number and address for people to contact you for appointments. In the beginning you will typically only be seeing a few clients per week,so you will be able to build your online presence overtime. In fact, I have a friend who works part time at her office specializing in sugaring, bringing in over $40,000 per year and only uses her Yelp and Facebook page to advertise her contact information and hours. She has not created a website yet.

If you have an excellent spa up in the woods somewhere with raving reviews about your signature pre and post pregnancy massages on Yelp and a high ranking website on Google for your specific keywords, you will most likely have as much business as you can handle. And the fact that you are not in a prime location in town doesn't matter as much because people easily found you online. They are willing to drive to you because you offer specifically what they are looking for.

In the beauty industry, there is more emphasis on quality of service and personal connection than on your actual physical location. That's why clients kept coming back to me month after month for massages, even though my spa music didn't always drown out the neighboring aerobics class or a crying baby in the nursery. I offered an excellent massage that was customized to their specific needs and I made a personal connection with them that couldn't be replaced going somewhere else.

When I first opened up Acomoclitic Studio, I chose an area that was near a developing outdoor mall. My plan was to rent the 500 square foot office for a year, build up a client base and then move into the mall. After a year of building my business, I already had a full schedule where I was located. If I moved into the mall, I would gain more exposure, but I couldn't take in more clients without hiring another esthetician. The earnings I would make after paying the higher rent plus the employee didn't make sense. I could make more money and have less stress staying where I was. Luckily, it turned out that another room in my building opened up that linked into my current space, so I was able to add another 300 square foot treatment room. With expanded hours and hiring more employees, I was able to increase revenue in my current location without a drastic increase in rent. Plus my brick and mortar location didn't affect my online product business one iota.

When putting together your business plan, evaluate your location and find something that works for you. But don't get hung up on it being perfect, especially right from the beginning. My philosophy is, start small with lower costs and as you build your client base, you can improve on your location. This is specifically related to estheticians and massage therapists. I can't speak for other industries. I have seen one too many people in my industry suffer because they picked a space too large or too expensive for them. Try to find something around $400 per month. You don't want all your hard earned money simply going to pay for the space you are in.

Some things to consider when choosing a location:

Cost per square foot: Many office spaces are labeled on the price per square foot which by the sounds of it, always makes it seem really cheap. Like $3.50 per square foot. But once you add up the total cost of everything, it usually isn't as affordable as it sounds. When inquiring about properties, ask them to tell you the exact amount you are going to be required to pay for rent every month rather than the square foot price. This is what I always did to make sure I wasn't miscalculating the costs.

CAM charges: There are always extra charges besides the base rent that need to be considered into your business plan. Sometimes CAM (Common Area Maintenance) charges can jump your rent by $200 or $300 per month, so you definitely want to make sure to find out what they are going to be. Some landlords can be rather sly about giving you exact figures on this, but if you keep asking the right questions you can gather a clear idea on of how much to estimate. CAM charges usually include garbage, water, electricity, snow removal and possibly improvements to the property like paving the parking lot or replacing the roof. The costs can vary from month to month and year to year, but the landlord should still be able to provide a reasonable estimate for you so you aren't blindsided by unexpected bills.

Utility costs: A lot of times these will be in the CAM charges and other times, these will be separate. Especially things like phone and internet.

***What you are responsible for and what the landlord is
responsible for:*** All of the details should be listed out in the lease
agreement; however, remember that any contract is negotiable. If
you try to negotiate on some of the terms and the landlord doesn't
budge, it may be worth getting a lawyer involved. It's always better
to come to terms prior to signing the lease because after you are
under contract it is difficult to make any changes. Sometimes this
can protect you from additional costs and other times, it can cost
you.

Unfortunately, I found out the hard way on a few of the
terms in my lease for Acomoclitic. For instance, my landlord
charged a $100 per day late charge fee. Even though I signed the
lease with the full intention of never being a day late on my rent,
there were times that I have made mistakes and had to pay a
huge fee. I didn't like this term when signing the lease, but I didn't
take any measures to negotiate with the landlord on a lower
penalty, a grace period or exceptions for holidays or weekends
when falling on the 1st of the month.

Another example is that the landlord was responsible for
the Air Conditioning (AC) and heating in my building. This seemed
great considering he would pay for any maintenance, repairs or
replacements. But it turned out the furnace and air conditioning
unit were aged and could not function at full capacity. In fact, on
really hot days, the AC breaker would switch off and we couldn't
switch it back on right away. It would usually take about 20-30
minutes before we could switch it back. This was causing the
treatment rooms to be extremely uncomfortable on some of those
hot Colorado summer days. Not only were the customers and
technicians uncomfortable, the wax or sugar would not work
properly and the laser would shut off from overheating.

Since this was a cost the landlord was responsible for, he
was determined not to pay any more than needed, and some
summers there wasn't any maintenance done such as cleaning or
replacing the filter.

It's hard to look back and know for sure what I could have
done differently. At least I could have asked him to add into the

lease that the space needed to be maintained at 70-75 degrees at all times. I could have asked more questions pertaining to the AC and heating system prior to leasing the space. Once I discovered how old they were and how little maintenance had been done, I could have requested that the units be replaced prior to moving into the space and make sure that it was written into the lease before signing.

Ultimately, I had to talk the landlord into letting me replace the systems at a cost of $4,400 since he was only willing to do basic maintenance on them which wasn't solving the issue. That summer was the first in 7 years that we had comfortable temperatures in the treatment rooms, even on over 100 degree days. It was so much better. And I can't even calculate how much business we lost because new clients didn't have a great experience and repeat clients were frustrated with the laser shutting off mid-service and sometimes having to reschedule if the laser wouldn't come back on. Plus, all the referrals they would have sent our way that were lost. However, clients can be won over even when circumstances are not perfect, like my massage clients having to deal with loud, unrelaxing sounds during their treatments at the women's fitness center. Luckily, it didn't damage business altogether, but I'm sure it had a cost, which made paying for the new AC and furnace a no brainer, even though the landlord should have paid for it.

So make sure to read all the details of the lease and be sure to negotiate anything that you have questions on. Learn from my mistakes. It would be helpful to get someone else to help you with this too, like a lawyer or someone with experience. And, as a general rule, at least ask for any changes you deem necessary to the contract.

_Insurance costs__:_ For basic esthetics and massage therapy insurance, I have found ABMP and ASCP are very reasonable and cover a lot. If you have employees or subcontractors, you can require them to pay for their own insurance. Make sure the insurance covers all the services you offer.

Once I added laser hair removal, I had to get a different insurance and it got much more expensive. I paid over $600 per month in insurance costs. In order to be insured for laser hair removal in Colorado, I needed a Medical Director which was an additional $1000 per month. Every state and county can have different regulations for your industry. This may change as laws change for licensing and certification, and as new services with new products and equipment are invented.

There are different types of insurance. One is for liability. Another to cover the building and equipment. For the laser, I had a separate insurance to cover the laser machine. Both my Medical Director and landlord were added to my insurance which didn't affect the cost.

You can ask for quotes from a few different companies to see what is the best deal and what covers the most before deciding on which one you want.

Understanding what your insurance covers and what it doesn't: I knew a Chiropractor who had a flood in his office space and it damaged quite a few things and he closed for business until the place was back in order. His insurance didn't cover any of the damage or lost business. He told me he regretted not getting insurance to cover flooding but he hadn't thoroughly looked through what his insurance covered and what it didn't cover. He assumed that it would cover costs incurred from floods. If you are leasing a space, there may also be areas of the building that are covered under the landlord's insurance. Paying for insurance is always a gamble since you never know if you are really going to need it, but for many businesses, insurance can come to the rescue in a dreadful circumstance. If you don't have it, it could be very costly and could in fact take down your entire business. As entrepreneurs, we are natural risk takers, but once you have a good business established, proper insurance is recommended and may even be mandated if you are leasing a space or equipment.

Zoning Laws: Acomoclitic Studio is located in an area that has strict city guidelines for signage. I was not having making progress getting permits for the signs I wanted to put up, so I finally put them up regardless of the permits. There could come a day when the zoning department comes by and asks me to take them down, fine me or make me pay for the permits, but I was willing to take this risk. The signs have been up for nearly a year now and I have not had anyone from zoning contact me. Because I feel that the signs are not obtrusive, I believe I would have an easier time getting permits now that they are up. This was a gamble I was willing to take, but ultimately it's best to abide by the zoning laws.

If you are going to work out of your home you will want to find out what the guidelines are for home businesses in your area. One massage therapist I know who worked out of her house couldn't post a sign in her yard, so she put advertising on her car and parked it in her driveway. That was an easy way around zoning. If you are allowed to put a sign up in your yard, it could be a great way to attract regular customers, since most likely they live or work close by making it easy to get to you for appointments. Zoning can sometimes seem really complicated, so if you are really uncertain about where to start, visit your local office and bring all your questions. If you are still uncertain about things or believe the information you got might be incorrect, speak to someone else in that office. I had a friend who worked in zoning and she said she was always willing to answer any questions and even give advice on how to accomplish whatever it was people were looking to do within the legal parameters. Hopefully you will find a friendly face at your local zoning office like my friend.

Chapter 2: Branding Yourself

Once you know your niche, branding yourself will be easier than ever before. Branding for a 'general' spa can be very challenging and I personally find it rather boring. When you have a niche, it can be really fun and sometimes funny to come up with ideas to brand yourself.

For quite awhile, I used a hairless cat as part of our branding. People enjoyed our sense of humor to use a 'hairless kitty' to market our most popular service. Unfortunately the cat we were using belonged to one of the employees. The cat died and she asked me not to use him for marketing purposes any longer.

The more specific you are in your branding, the easier it is for people to remember and the easier it is to brand yourself. There are whole books and classes on branding. There are people who are experts at branding. However, you don't have to pay someone else to brand your business. Let your imagination work for you and think of things you like. Especially if you are going to be the only service provider in your business, your brand can really be like a personal statement of yourself. Choose a look and feel that represents you.

If you do have a vision of franchising your business some day, the more thought you put into your brand, the easier it will be to multiply it. And the more valuable it will be because since the day you opened, you were marketing your specific brand.

Knowing your niche really does save time with your branding. For example, let's say you want your niche to be reflexology for people with allergies. Doesn't that make creating your business card so much more simple? I immediately think of a foot shape since it is commonly used to represent reflexology and a sniffling nose to represent an allergic reaction. What about "Kick Your Allergies Good-Bye" with a foot kicking a Kleenex? The business name could be "Relief-flexology". Next to your name you can put your title as 'Reflexologist'. Your website could be www.relief-flexology.com. I just came up with this in a few minutes. Imagine if you spent a few hours brainstorming. You could come up with some clever ideas on how you want to brand yourself starting with a business card.

When coming up with your own brand, here are some things to think about that you could incorporate:

1. your name
2. your website
3. your email address
4. your phone number--You could use a special number saying something like 303-WAX-LEGS
5. your street address--Alameda Laser
6. town/city/name of area--Cherry Creek Acne Facials
7. colors
8. logo
9. mission statement
10. tagline
11. look or feel you want to portray

When I was looking for a logo to use for Acomoclitic, I hired a graphic person to help me come up with something. It would have worked out well, if I was happy with one of the first few designs he showed me. Unfortunately, I wasn't and I kept giving him more and more chances to 'get it right'. When all was said and done, I told him it didn't seem like we were on the same page and I was going to find someone else to design it. It still costed me nearly $2,000 for his time. I ended up finding my logo on LogoYes.com and as soon as I saw it, I knew it was the right one. I liked that program so much, I ended up choosing my Vadazzle logo from that site as well. What I love about most of Logoyes designs is that they are simple. Our crown has been easy to embroider on our uniforms, put up as a big sticker on our reception wall, and easy to recognize. It's very user friendly and memorable. The Vadazzle logo has a similar shape to one of our popular sparkly gem designs and also looks like a V. It's perfect!

Another idea is using a company like Vistaprint which offers a variety of marketing materials with the same pattern once you choose one. One of my esthetician friends used Vistaprint and chose one of their designs that was red and black. She was able to get her business cards and brochures and website all with that specific look and feel. She then used those colors to decorate her office. Her brand was easily recognizable and made a lasting impression.

Overall, branding is definitely important for you to spend some time on. It doesn't have to be difficult. In fact, usually the simpler the better because people will be able to notice it and remember it.

After I had been in business for a couple years, I hired a guy who had a background in putting together branding guides. Primarily this guide was clarifying colors, fonts, logos, and even the tone of the pictures used. This branding guide was helpful because when using a variety of media to advertise, each company had their own graphic person. Each person had their own style and could easily create an ad that looked very different from our brand. By having a guide for the font styles and colors, it really helped. Even when I would get a proof that was not aligned with the guide, I was easily able to communicate with the graphic person what changes needed to be made by referring to the branding guide. I used this guide for our brochures, for our signs, for every print ad and online ads, mailers, newsletters, and our webpages.

Even though this type of branding is important and helpful in getting clients to recognize your logo or ads in various media, there is more to a brand than black and white. What I mean is that your brand has a lot to do with the customer experience. How does your customer feel at your spa? This feeling can be translated into the fonts and colors but there are other factors. For instance, the way your company answers the phone, sets appointments, what their experience is like when at your shop or on your website, what the colors and style is of your space, etc. Most likely your brand will match your personal style especially if you are the main person doing the services or even answering the calls. What is it that you personally offer? One of the things I often got complimented on when I was a massage therapist was a nice bedside manner. My clients felt safe, cared for and listened to. They were able to relax in my presence. I have carried over some of that feeling to Acomoclitic. My mission statement actually says 'safe and comfortable place' because it was important for me to give clients that type of atmosphere for such an intimate service. Since I have opened, I have always hired estheticians who also were able to portray this type of feeling. I want the clients to take a breath of relief when they meet their esthetician since new clients usually come in a little apprehensive. When our reviews describe the staff as 'calming or easy going' I know that my brand is working.

I would recommend spending some time contemplating and investigating what type of 'feeling' you want your brand to be. It really helps having a solid description. I have found that by knowing my brand it has made it easier to make decisions such as who to hire or what type of interior decorating to go with. If you open your business with one idea, don't be afraid to change it after a couple years if your clients are giving you feedback that doesn't fit with your original idea. When I first opened my business, I went with a more relaxed, beachy look and feel. It was my first decorator who was also a client who helped me change my look and bring in the black and silver with my gold. When she recommended painting one of the walls of our reception black I was taken back. The thing was is that my clients were getting a more sexy, sleek look from my business and services, especially with the nude black and white photos I was already using. After I redid the floors and walls of the space, I started to incorporate black and silver into my brand and I got rid of the turquoise. The gold stayed the same. I felt like this was a good move because it did match more of what the clients were experiencing anyway and now I had the colors to go along with that feeling.

One time I was advertising in a newspaper and they sent me a proof that I disapproved of but because they were on a time crunch, they ran the ad without my approval. The ad was so different from my brand I was very frustrated. After putting so much time and energy into my brand and having something I really liked, I hated that this ad ran that totally botched it up. I made a big deal about my disappointment to the newspaper and when the agent and his boss came over to meet with me, I broke down in tears telling them how the ad didn't represent my company. Maybe it was that time of month, but whatever it was, it did make me realize how much I loved my brand and wanted to protect it.

As far as proofing your ads, one tip I got was to always check the phone number, address and website. It's easy to overlook. Luckily I haven't had any ad printed with the wrong phone number yet, but one time I did have a bunch of business cards printed with the wrong number since I didn't double check it was correct and they all ended up in the trash.

When you think of all the time and energy you put into creating your brand, there is value there. If you have a really great brand, you may end up selling your brand to others to use. If you do have future plans to franchise or sell your brand, you may not want to name your business after yourself, your street or your town. Another thing to think about in the larger picture, is if you ever want to open up more locations, the simpler your brand is, the easier it is to duplicate. So if you do have a vision for multiple locations in your future, keep that in mind because that will affect your brand.

Keeping a simple menu of services is helpful as well because if you do start another location, you will need to invest in all the various products and equipment needed to perform all your services, plus more extensive training when hiring staff. The less you offer, the less expensive it is to start another location.

Awhile ago, I did experiment with selling the Acomoclitic brand to a couple other estheticians who wanted to start up Acomoclitic Studios. I'm glad I tried it, but ultimately it didn't end up working out. I was not fully prepared and didn't have a clear plan. One of the hurdles I faced was that they did not have the capital to purchase all of the lasers, equipment and products they would have needed to match all of the services and products I was selling. Even as specialized as I was with Acomoclitic, I still had too much going on to make it profitable to duplicate. I also found that I was spending more time and energy helping those two other businesses that was taking away from my focus on the main store. Looking back, I realized that I needed to be more prepared. There were additional expenses and bookkeeping costs, and I had a loss of business from the main store when clients went to the new locations. I had expected this to happen but wasn't prepared for the loss in revenues. The deal ended up being too costly to make it worthwhile so I made the decision to pull out. The positive that came out of that situation is that each of those estheticians created their own unique company which was easier having already had a foundation to start from since they had opened with my brand and my consulting. They are still in business to this day and doing well, offering different services and products than I offered. They have more freedom to create their own brand. I am proud that I was a part of their accomplishments, which shows that one of my passions is helping others create and be successful in this industry.

Whether you are thinking big or small, putting some thought and care into your brand from the beginning will increase your chance of success. If you are already in business, perhaps you have been in business for years at this point, you may have a brand but never really took time to sculpt it or describe it. If you take some time today, this week or this month to marinate in how you would describe your brand, even asking your clients for their feedback, you can create some needed clarity. You will find that once you have that clarity, it gives you renewed energy. You also can communicate your brand so much easier. It won't be so hard to come up with promotions or newsletters or even how to decorate your space and what to wear to work. You can start letting go of the services or things that aren't congruent with your brand. It makes it easier for you to pick what classes or trainings you might want to take. It helps you decide what things are complimenting growing your business and which things may be distracting from growing your business.

Compare this process to redecorating a room in your home that has quite a bit of red and brown but also some gold, green and blue. It looks nice and there is a cozy feeling to it, but it's one of those rooms that you have never really put much thought into. You bought things that you liked or perhaps were given some items that filled the space. One day you decide that you really like the red and brown together and want that to stand out. Now that you have made that decision, it has you start making all sorts of changes to the room so that those two colors really pop out and aren't muffled by the other colors. After you have things rearranged in the room, and most likely a handful of things set aside to sell or giveaway, you may even bring some new items into the space that accentuate your new look. After a couple years, you may even do another 'look over' to make sure your room hasn't been cluttered up again by things that take away the focus from your brown and red theme.

A similar approach is required with your business to keep a strong, healthy brand. Since you are the creator of your company, only you can do this, even though the clients are the ones that will reinforce it through word of mouth, you can initiate what you want them to say to their friends about your business by having clarity yourself.

Once you have a good idea of your brand then it's time to start marketing. And because you took time to really think about your niche and branding, it makes marketing much easier.

Chapter 3: Marketing Your Niche

Marketing has ended up being one of the most important skills I have developed. When building your business, I highly recommend learning marketing. I was at a business class earlier this year and one of the speakers came out on stage and asked everyone, "What business are you in?" and everyone started shouting out their unique businesses when the speaker interrupted and said, "If you didn't say marketing, you won't be successful." Being in any business requires marketing because until people know how to find you, you have no business.

Marketing is anything that can result in a sale to a new client or repeat client. Here are some tools and ideas that I have used and you might consider using for your marketing purposes:

- brochures
- business cards
- flyers
- mailers
- postcards
- networking: luncheons, meetup groups, leads groups, networking functions, charities, clubs, committees, chamber events
- newspaper
- magazines
- groupon
- newsletter
- e-newsletter
- website
- search engine optimization (SEO)
- referral programs for clients and other businesses
- open house
- free gift with purchase
- Bring a friend and get a discount
- door to door
- car flyers

- bulletin boards
- bathrooms
- gyms
- car magnets
- bumper stickers
- pens
- radio
- TV
- Billboards
- Bus stop Ads
- Better Business Bureau
- Joining your local chamber
- signs
- banners

Marketing is the only way that your business is going to grow. One thing I did that worked well was to choose a different marketing approach for each year. Sometimes I chose things to stretch my comfort zone because I learned from T Harv Eker that when you expand your comfort zone, you expand your money zone.

My first year starting my massage business, I grew primarily through an add in a local mailer offering a $39 hour massage. I also offered free 15 minute chair massages to the women at the gym. After the free session, I asked if they would like to make an appointment for an hour massage at a discounted price of $39. The next year, I opened up another office at a chiropractor's, so I was able to market to his clientele. He happened to be a brand new business, so he offered a massage deal in some local magazines to get people into his office in hopes that they would also need chiropractic services. I didn't even have to pay for the ads but I did pay him a commission on my income instead of a flat monthly rent.

When I bought the Day Spa in Littleton, the previous owner had always done ads in a coupon mailer and had success with bringing in new clients as well as return clients who knew to look for her regular coupons. I kept doing those. The next year, I bought a full page ad in a phone book, and it included eight coupons in the back of the phone book that people could pull out to use at the spa.

As you can tell by my efforts in these early years, things have changed quite a bit in marketing. Phonebooks? What are those? That is another good reason to continuously try out new marketing ideas so you aren't left behind in the dust as other businesses grab up all the new business by staying with the trends of where people are looking and searching for spa services.

When Groupon first came out, I gave it a go and had great success. That was the best time to do it because it was a brand new concept and I was able to make a huge amount of money in a very short period of time. Now Groupon has changed so the funds trickle in but back then was the bomb! I remember making over $30,000 in a week on a laser promotion! Since you can't take advantage of Groupon like you could in the very beginning, I won't go into detail about it since you can't apply the same strategy today. The only thing I will say is that if you see or hear about a new type of marketing, be open to exploring it. I'm sure many estheticians and massage therapists in that time didn't even open their door to the Groupon marketing person and lost a huge opportunity to expand their business. I was open to learning about the new advertising and I wasn't scared to give it go. In fact, I was more confident in working with them because even though I had to give a significant discount, I was guaranteed new clients compared to other types of advertising that gave absolutely no guarantees. As Groupon wisened up to how they ran their company, I also wisened up to what types of services and discounts were the most beneficial to my bottom line. I kept doing Groupon type marketing up until I sold Acomoclitic and the new owner continued to use Groupon as well.

One tried and true marketing strategy that I believe will always work in our industry is networking. When I opened Acomoclitic Studio, I decided to push myself by going to networking groups. I was shy at first but as I did more, I got better at socializing and promoting my new business. Because I wasn't super busy with clients yet, I had plenty of time to attend a lot of events. I went to the Chamber events, Better Business Bureau events, and then I was invited to a handful of leads groups as a guest. I started going to some charity events to network. From there I was invited to other social groups, some that were for men and women but my favorite ones were women only, like Denver Divas.

I met a lot of people at these events. I was able to do some trades with the other business people I met that helped grow my business. For instance, one guy traded me ad space in his magazine for laser hair removal on his back. I also traded with a lady who was a relationship coach to advertise my services to her email list. I met another gal who did spray tans and for awhile she would come to my studio and do spray tans for my customers. Eventually she got so busy, she trained me on how to do it, sold me a spray gun and tent, and then I bought the spray tan solution from her as needed. I really grew to love networking even though I was nervous about it in the beginning. Not only did it help market my new business, but I also made some life long friends. As I got busier, I didn't have time to go to as many events but it was a great way to do marketing and it was tons of fun!

The nice thing about having a niche, is that when you are out networking, you will be more memorable to the people you meet. For example, if you meet a hair stylists and they tell you they are a hair stylist you will likely forget them or what they do. But if you met a hair stylist who tells you they specialize in hair extensions, or are the expert in hair extensions, it's easier to remember, especially if you notice their long beautiful natural looking hair extensions they are wearing. And then if they take it a step further and say "I specialize in hair extensions for people who have short hair and want long hair" and they hand you a business card that has a before and after photo of someone with short hair and then the after photo shows the same person with gorgeous long hair, you are much more likely to remember this person and what they do. Visual is memorable. It's very specific and unique. Business cards are a must when you are out networking. And it's important to be gathering other people's business cards as well, so you can keep in touch with them.

During the first years of growing Acomoclitic, I also used craigslist ads which brought in new customers every week. The next year I decided to hire someone to do Search Engine Optimization (SEO) for me. Every year, I usually had one big emphasis with my marketing even though I did some other things too. I tried to change up my main focus every year. I figured that way I was reaching a new audience that I may not have reached through previous efforts.

In 2013 my word was PERSISTENCE. I like having a word each year because it keeps me focused. In fact, in 2013 I made a goal to jump from $350k per year to $500k per year which I knew would require some additional marketing (and persistence). I went gangbusters and spent an additional $30,000 in marketing by hiring an SEO company, did some expensive postcard advertising, went on Colorado Best TV show, advertised in the Westword, put on an Open House, sent out a couple mailers to our clients, hired a virtual assistant to contact all our clients on facebook individually (if they were on there) and sent our clients an individual email asking for updated contact information with an incentive.

Even though I exceeded my goal of $500k which I couldn't have done without the additional advertising, it seemed like the highest return came from our Yelp page (which is free), our e-newsletter which cost $100 a month with Constant Contact, our online store which is free with our scheduling system, referrals which we pay our clients $10 in credit for, print materials like brochures and business cards, and our website maintenance and updates. All of these things had a much higher return on investment than the more expensive avenues. I loved when clients came in from Yelp because of all the positive reviews, they were more comfortable right from the get go. I also noticed this with clients who were personally referred by someone. It seemed like they already knew me and felt comfortable with me, so it took less work to 'win them over' so to speak. I discovered that oftentimes it was the least expensive things I did that brought in the most clients and the most loyal clients.

The next year I made a goal to grow to $750k but this time I decided to invest more into the staff and clients which was a new marketing strategy I had not tried before. I lowered my budget for outside marketing to $1,000 per month which was a drastic drop from 2013 but I did believe that the previous years efforts would overflow into 2013. My plan for 2014 was to market with a different approach, more of an internal marketing strategy. I was fortunate to have employees that had worked for me for a few years or more, and I wanted to keep them. One way I invested in my staff was by bringing in additional sales training, product knowledge, service training and increasing their pay and benefits. I wanted my staff to feel really special. I wanted them to feel proud of their expertise and also be challenged to learn more and grow. By improving their sales skills and client retention, the customers would ultimately be more pampered with our products and services on a regular basis, which would reflect in higher revenues. I was hoping that by improving my staff experience, it would be relayed to the clients with an attractive vibe. I changed the hours of operation which resulted in less gaps during the day which the estheticians preferred. My hope was that the handful of regular clients the change affected would be able to find another day and time that worked within the new hours. I continued with the low cost marketing that worked well the year before, and invested more in marketing to our client list. My goal was to improve the customer experience.

The word I chose for 2014 was EFFICIENCY. As the word EFFICIENCY stayed front and center in my mind throughout the year, it helped me make adjustments and decisions that produced positive results. I gave efficiency priority over other things which resulted in less frivolous spending and higher profits, less wasted hours and increased productivity, moving from complicated to simple, and less clutter. If you are reading this book and deciding to narrow your business down to a specific niche, feel free to steal this word. It would be a good one while you are transitioning your business into a specific niche.

When it comes to marketing, efficiency is important. Every dollar you spend you should at least gain $3 back. That's just a general rule of thumb. But I tell you, some of the best marketing is word of mouth and free stuff like blogging, social media, being listed in directories such as Yelp and putting ads on craigslist. Another high return item is a monthly email to your client list. This is a great way to keep in touch with them and let them know what is going on at your spa. It's also an easy place to educate clients on new services or products. Sometimes we forget that not everyone knows what exfoliation is, or what Vitamin A does for the skin, or what a hot stone massage is. Doing an article or a video in your newsletter is one way to promote your services simply by educating your customers on what they are. Chapter 5 goes more in depth about educating the public but this is an important part of marketing. Especially if you have a product or service that is awesome but very few people have heard of or understand the benefits of.

Once I had staff doing all of the services and a call center taking the calls, I could step away from the business as much or as little as I wanted. I found that even when I would return from vacations, I would be spending the majority of my time on marketing efforts. Marketing has become my all time favorite thing! There are a gazillion strategies out there and that is why I do find that having one main focus each year helps. That way you really get to give it a full effort. If you are dabbling around with a bunch of different things but not able to give each one a true opportunity to show the results, it's hard to track what marketing efforts are working and which ones aren't. Plus, I find it drains my energy...and could drain your checking account if you are trying too many at the same time. The other reason I liked this strategy is because I was constantly being approached by advertising companies and when I was clear on what my budget was and what strategies I was doing that year, I was more decisive in which ones I did and which ones I said no to. Occasionally I would be interested in one of the advertising options a sales person would bring me but instead of signing up right then, I would tell them it wasn't in the budget this year, but I would like to discuss it with them the following year.

Whatever marketing you choose, make note of how much it costs you and what your return on investment is. Take time to narrow down to the marketing that is working the best for you and eliminate the rest. Don't keep doing something if the return is not there. When I first started into this industry, phonebooks were a great way to gain clients. I had a phone number that tracked the calls from the phonebook listing and one year I only had three calls the entire year and two were from advertisers, so it was an easy decision not to renew my listing. As more people were finding me online, I chose to invest more money into my online presence. Be open to exploring new ways of marketing and new trends. If your revenues are staying the same from year to year, or especially if they start going down, don't be afraid to stop what you are doing and try something new.

Things to consider with marketing:
  1. **Who is your target market?** This question is easily answered if your niche is your target market, such as golfers, pregnant women or grooms. If your niche is a service, then take some time to picture who those people are that want that type of service. Look at the map and decide what areas (neighborhoods, towns, cities) your

target market is in.

2. **Who are your ideal clients?** One simple answer is people who can afford your services. But you can be as specific as you want beyond that. In fact, the more specific you are, the easier it will be for you to find those ideal clients and for them to find you. It is highly recommended and worthwhile to spend some serious focus on describing your ideal client in detail. You will find that by doing this, you will be very clear on where and how to market your business and will be much more successful in finding these clients. Actually, your ideal clients may not be people who can afford your services, let's say if your niche is geared towards children or minors, or paid by insurance. Another niche you may have could be offering services to people who don't pay for the service. Perhaps you make your money through donations from others so you can give away free services to underprivileged people in your niche i.e. acne treatments for troubled teens, energy work for people detoxing off drugs, craniosacral therapy for children with Tourette's. If you do this, you would want to set up your company as a Non Profit for additional tax benefits and so people who donate can also have tax incentives.

3. **How are you going to track results?** Having a system for tracking your marketing efforts is really helpful to know which ones to keep doing and which ones to stop doing. The main thing you need to track is how new clients are finding you since gaining a new client is usually more expensive than retaining a current client. For marketing to your current clients, you can track things like client retention, who opens your emails, who clips coupons, who's participating in referral programs, upsells or add on services, re-booking, products bought, etc. There are quite a few really helpful scheduling software systems for massage therapists and estheticians that have all the capabilities for tracking these things and pulling reports. I worked with a business coach who was adamant that I

give her specific numbers on how much a marketing effort cost and how much money I made from it. It was hard for me at first because I had not created a habit of tracking those things in detail. Once I took the time to figure out the numbers, it was extremely helpful in seeing what worked and what didn't, where before I would go with more of a gut feeling but didn't have the hard facts to back it up.

4. **What fits your personality?** Each person is going to be drawn to different types of marketing based on their personality. Some forms of advertisement will be more fun or easier for you than others. I pushed myself from being shy in networking situations to being more outgoing, but in the beginning, you may want to start with marketing that is easy for you to get started with. Is Facebook your thing? Is putting on an open house or event your thing? Is blogging your thing? Is Youtube videos your thing? What feels comfortable for you? This is a good place to start because it won't feel like you are spending so much energy if it is a form of marketing that you enjoy.

5. **What areas do you want to stretch yourself in?** As your business grows, look outside of your comfort zone for some new ways of marketing. This could be as simple as doubling your google adwords budget, or as wild as dressing up in a large hand costume (that has your massage business name on it) at a parade and passing out coupons with suckers. If you let your imagination go and think outside the box, you could come up with some unusual ways to attract attention to your business. Some efforts will be more effective than others but don't be afraid to try some new things and see what happens.

6. **What can you do yourself?** In the beginning, you have more time and energy to spend on marketing and can do a lot of it yourself. As you get busy with customers, you have less time. If you want to keep growing your business, you will either be spending time on marketing that you could be with clients, or you can spend some of your hard earned

money to put into marketing. Then if you follow in my footsteps and hire people to do the services, you can go back to doing more marketing yourself. The more involved you are in the marketing, the easier it is for you to track the success.

7. **What do you need to contract out (or utilize trades)?** Be open to doing trades for marketing purposes. Some ideas are: giving someone who writes articles a free product or service in exchange for writing an article about your niche business, promoting someone else's business in your e-newsletter in exchange for them promoting your business to their email list, trading banner advertisements on each others websites, trading print ads for services, trading services with clients to help at booths, etc. You won't always be able to trade, so have a budget which could be a dollar amount or a percentage of sales that you spend on marketing. And of course you don't want to spend that money without it giving you business in return, so spend that money wisely.

8. **What are your goals?** The clearer you are on your goals, the more confident you will be in knowing how much time, money and energy to put into marketing efforts. If you are only wanting to grow your business to 3 clients per day then your marketing will be much different compared to someone growing their business to support three full time reflexologists. If you want your product revenues to be 50% of your overall sales, your marketing will be much different than someone who only plans on 5% of their overall sales coming from products. Goals will help guide you. Business is fluid and there is not a straight line to meeting your goals, but having them will give you an understanding of how much marketing is needed to reach them.

Chapter 4: Becoming the Best

Becoming the best is where your business really starts to become FUN! We've all heard the saying 'Jack of all trades but master of none' right? No matter how great you think you are right now at doing a massage or a facial, it's nothing compared to how great you will be once you pick a niche to specialize in and do that service all day every day. When I was doing 6-8 massages per day on all sorts of different types of clients, I was good but not great! I wasn't specialized in any specific body type or massage technique. When I started doing facials, I was working on all types of skin and didn't have expertise in anything specific. When starting out into this industry, it's great to gain some experience working on a variety of clients but with such a vast amount of niches to choose from, don't wait too long before narrowing in on your chosen niche. The sooner you choose your niche, the sooner you can become the best!

Keys to Becoming the Best

> **Practise.** The more you do what you want to specialize in, the better you become. The best way to get practise is to start marketing yourself for your new 'niche' to bring in more clients to work on. You can also offer what you do to some of your friends and family at a discount. The more practise you have, the more you are branding yourself for what you are offering, whether it is pregnancy massage, reflexology for allergies or ingrown hair treatments. In the beginning, don't be afraid to offer your niche service for free or a great discount so you can gain practise and exposure. For instance, if you want to specialize in massage for the elderly, see if you can do free hand or foot massages at the local nursing home. If you want to do pre-natal massage, see if your obstetrician would let you set up free chair massage in their waiting room for their patients to make their wait time more enjoyable. By practising more and more on your chosen clientele, you will learn more than any book will ever teach you. Plus, you

will start gaining the exposure to your target market which opens up opportunities for new clients and new business.

- ➢ *Educate yourself.* NEVER EVER get to a point that you feel like no one knows better than you or has anything to offer you. That is when you will fall behind the trends. Stay up to date on the latest and greatest. Get educated on every new product, equipment or unique technique that you come across relating to your niche. Be open to exploring new ways of doing things. Try things out on yourself or on your close friends to see if it's something you want to incorporate into your business. If you like it, practise using it on your clients and get their feedback while at the same time getting better at using the new technique or familiarizing yourself with a new product. There is a lot of free education online that you can take advantage of. If you spent one hour a day studying your field of expertise, imagine how much better you will become. It can be as easy as watching a couple youtube videos. If you are specializing in working on people with a certain disease, keep studying that disease. Ask a lot of questions. Be open to learning new information or even conflicting information. The more familiar you are with your niche, the better you will become and soon you will be the best!

- ➢ *Sell yourself as the best* at what you specialize in. Don't be afraid to say that you are the best. There is no one else who does what you do the way that you do it and as much as you do it, so that makes you the specialist. Put on your business card "Expert" or "Specializing in..." or "Specialist". Highlight your expertise. You can start doing this before you become as great as you want to become because it will help you get there faster. By promoting yourself as the expert, it gives you confidence and posture. If you are like me, you will keep getting better at what you do everyday. Perhaps the first year in your niche, you weren't as much of an expert as you are after 5 years. That's okay. You can still advertise yourself as the expert now. You don't have to wait 5 years. Even when I hired staff to work for me, I named them a specialist in Brazilian hair removal right from the beginning. After going through my training, they were already much more experienced and knowledgeable than most estheticians are on Brazilians, so I felt I had discretion doing this, even though I knew that it would take about six months to a year for them to gain the experience to be truly one of the best around. I felt that after I had done a thousand Brazilians, I was an expert because by that time I had worked on such a variety of different hair types, skin types, body types and sensitivities, I had mastered the skill. I knew how to get even the toughest hair out of the most sensitive person with success. By that time I still had not tried sugaring, so that was a whole new level of expertise that came later. And I can almost guarantee that as you start diving into a niche area, you will go through layers of expanding your skills. If you are afraid of not having enough variety, just wait. You will be shocked at how much variety you can find in any chosen niche and you may find yourself choosing to narrow down even more. For instance, prior to opening Acomoclitic, my business plan was to offer full body wax and laser, spray tanning and brow and lash tinting which was very narrowed down after owning a Day Spa where we offered waaaayyyy more services than that. After only a short time, I was adding in a machine to get rid of skin tags, an LED machine to treat stretch marks, photofacials, microdermabrasion, microneedling, vadazzle, plus anal and vaginal bleaching. Besides the photofacial, all of these new services supported the Brazilian and the skin underneath. I had never even considered removing skin tags or stretchmarks prior to specializing in Brazilians. They were excellent add on services which I will discuss more in depth in Chapter 6.

➢ **Stay true to your niche.** It's easy to get off course in the beauty industry because of all the fun, new and exciting services and products that come out every season. It's also tempting when your clients are asking you "do you do botox? do you do nails? do you do massage?" It has you think...man I could make another $50 bucks if I offered those things. But actually it would start muffling with your brand. It will start having your clients not marketing for you the way you want them to. If you want to be known as the best Thai Massage Therapist or the best Hydra Facial Esthetician or the best Electrologist, you don't want to get too far off course with other services. Stay true to your niche so you can continue being the best and find sources that do the other services that you can refer to. If you are referring to someone often like for Botox or Massage, ask them for a finder's fee or a store credit that you can take advantage of. If you are referring people to buy a product, see if you can get a commission or if there is an affiliate program offered. For instance, if the product is sold on Amazon, you can become an Amazon affiliate and send your client the affiliate link so they can purchase it from there and you can get a kick back.

There are going to be certain services or products that clients ask you about that you will want to incorporate. These are those trends that you don't want to miss out on. For instance, if you are a nail shop and haven't caught on to doing the Shellac nails, you are missing out on a lot of business and happy customers. This was a trend you wouldn't want to pass up if your niche is already in nails. But I wouldn't recommend incorporating it into your massage business. For me, adding in electrolysis and sugaring was a smart choice because it related to my niche of doing Brazilians. I ended up offering photofacials at Acomoclitic because the first machine I had to do hair removal also did photofacials. Looking back, I would have been just as well off, not offering photofacials. It was a distraction from my niche. It was one more thing to train the staff on and it took away from being known for hair removal.

For every new service or product you bring into sell, you have to consider all of the marketing that is going to go into selling it. Most products and services don't sell themselves. If you decide to bring in something new, run the numbers. Make sure it makes financial sense. Consider how many do you have to sell, to make a profit. How long will that take? Does that make sense, or would you be smarter to put that money into marketing the services or products you are already selling? As you can tell by the title of this book, in order to get rich, you have to stay true to your niche. As soon as you start diversifying, you lose your mojo.

Make it your goal to becoming the best in your chosen niche. Start visualizing yourself as being the best in your community and then your state and then the country and then the world. You may not even realize the potential right now because you haven't put in the time or focus necessary. By becoming a specialist you may even have a technique named after you like Ida Rolf creating Rolfing, or Bikram Choudhury creating Bikram Yoga. As you hone in your skill or your chosen target market, or whatever it is you choose as your niche, you are going to discover a whole new world of possibilities.

Depending on what area you choose to go into, you may be the only one who ever took the expertise to that level. You will be opening yourself up to discover needs that perhaps have never been met before. It's almost like you become a scientist. Let's say you choose to work on professional swimmers as an esthetician and massage therapist. A common theme is dryness of skin from the swimming pools' chlorinated water. You work on so many swimmers that you even start to notice what areas of the body are always dry. Or what common symptoms swimmers always complain about. Let's say you discover that a special essential oil has immediate results and your clients are all having similar experiences of relief when you use that essential oil on them. Maybe you end up concocting a body wrap that includes the essential oil along with some other ingredients you have found are wonderfully effective in resolving swimmer's issues. Imagine that swimmers started spreading the word about this wonderful solution and all the professional swimmers across the world were demanding this service. You can see how this could really become something big. There might be so much demand that you decide to sell the product already mixed up and ready to go for the swimmers to apply at home along with either disposable or reusable wrap and a special application stick (or something) so they could get the product on their back (if they didn't have anyone to help them). Now that it is something swimmers could apply for themselves at home, this could get popular amongst all swimmers (not just the professionals) and you could be selling this even to high school kids or young children who are having the same skin issue because of the pool water.

There's really no limit on how big this could get. As this product is spreading around, more swimmers are going to know about you which gives you so many more opportunities. How you decide to capitalize on that is up to you. Just to give you some ideas, you could write a book on proper skin care for swimmers. You could sell instructional DVDs on how to get the most out of using the body wrap. You could team up with a famous swimmer who endorses your product and do magazine ads in swimmers magazines, or sports magazines. You could end up getting a free pass to the Olympic games to give all the swimmers this special body wrap service who would also be paying you top dollar for it. You could create some other complimentary products such as a moisturizing body wash or shaving cream that has that same essential oil.

I hope this little example gives you some inspiration on why becoming the best in a very specialized niche is your key to success. I made it sound super easy too which it can be when there is demand, and at the same time, it does take some strategy and leg work. Putting together the at home kit for the swimmers could be a challenge. Especially while you are so busy doing services, when are you going to have time to put together these kits? That's why the passion is so important. When you have such a strong desire to help swimmers with their skin, you are driven and it won't feel like so much work compared to doing something you have no interest in. It also could take a year to get it all together even though you would like it to only take a week. And of course there are the costs associated with putting them together with no guarantee on how long it will take to sell them all. As you are faced with these decisions, it's important to keep strategizing, keep dreaming, keep writing down goals, keep focused, and minimize your risk by always starting small. I constantly encourage estheticians to start with what they have. It's so easy to go and spend thousands of dollars but when you are in the service business that means thousands of hours. And you have to ask yourself, do I want to work all those hours just to launch a new product perfectly from the get go, with no guarantee on how long it will take to get my money back? In the case of at home body wraps, you could just put 10 jars together, get 10 wraps, and don't even worry about how to help them get it on their back with a special apparatus. Since in the beginning you would probably be marketing this to local swimmers, you could set up a small table at the next swim meet and promote your services as well as the take home product. Maybe you sell out of the 10 jars and have to take orders for future ones. Maybe you only sell 1 or 2. And if you only sold two, you would be happy that you only made ten and didn't get carried away with making up 100.

Even though when creating a product that you know there is a huge need for, you will personally have to do the marketing to promote it, as well as influence the demand for it. For instance, since you were the 'scientist' who made this discovery, you will need to bring this information to light. It first starts with talking to your clients about it and letting them know that they aren't the only ones with this issue. That many swimmers suffer from the same thing and you have found that your services and products are helping. Then you could take it further with writing articles, or making videos, even taking before and after pictures and posting them on your website. Everything you do to educate people about what you have found as a problem and solution will start to create more demand and ultimately make you wealthier as people pay for your 'solutions'.

Let's get back to "Being the Best". That is what this chapter is about and ultimately is what this book is about. When you find your niche and start diving into it with practise and learning and growing your client base and making connections, it feels really great. Your confidence grows and grows. Your reputation all of sudden goes from 'she's an esthetician/massage therapist' to 'she's the best esthetician/massage therapist for _____'. Which is great because now people are out there spreading the word for you. What I want you to get from this chapter is that you have to decide first that you are going to be the best at your niche. It's not going to happen without you making that decision. Then you have to post it on your business cards and start proclaiming it. You may find that it feels a bit funny at first. Especially if you already have an established reputation as just being an esthetician or massage therapist without any unique niche business. Now all of a sudden you are telling your clients and others that you are the world's greatest at _____. What I have found is that even though it feels a bit awkward at first, it will quickly attract your niche business and it won't take very long for you to really feel like you are the best. I would guesstimate that in about six months you will be over any awkward feelings about proclaiming yourself as the best because you will have had enough experience and education by that point. From then on, it will be about perfecting your chosen skill.

Don't be afraid to try out some variations of techniques or products as you go along. This is all part of being a scientist. You may find some things don't work as well as others but if you never try it, you won't know. Keep investigating. Dive deeper and deeper into exploring. Your million dollar discovery could be around the bend.

Chapter 5: Educating the Public

Many of the tools I mentioned in the Marketing chapter are used to educate the public such as brochures and blogging. Educating the public is marketing and yet it is such an important part for people who choose a niche that I wanted to devote an entire chapter to the subject. Plus, this will be another way to set yourself up as the expert. Educating the public is one way to build trust. When it comes to people spending money, they want to trust they are getting something in return. You have information about resolving others' pain in a very specific way and in order for people to find you, they must learn about how the process works. People are naturally curious and at the same time very busy. Finding places and methods of educating people that fit their busy lifestyle is a challenge and yet when you are passionate and determined, it is actually quite fun and rewarding.

Here are a few methods that I have used:
- Radio talk shows
- Magazine Articles
- Online media and articles
- Brochures
- Short presentations at leads groups
- Presentations and talks (more lengthy)
- Podcasts
- Online Radio Shows
- Infomercials
- Youtube
- Google Hangout interviews
- Books
- Website
- Blogging
- Frequently Asked Questions (FAQs)
- Forums
- Online chat
- Recorded presentations
- Recorded interviews

- Social Media

One important thing to consider when you are educating the public is: who are you educating? who is your audience? and what is your purpose for educating them? I believe some of this comes naturally, but it is something I will point on. When you are excited about something and knowledgable about it, a lot of times you want to tell people everything you know but unless they are wanting to become an expert too, they probably aren't interested in so much detail. In this chapter I will focus on educating the public. In the last chapter, I will discuss more about educating your industry. Both of those audiences are going to be different and you will want to adjust your message based on your audience.

One tip to get the most response is to think about what the need is for your public. Or what is their 'pain' that you resolve. It is worth your energy to take a few moments to consider this. You could even ask some of your clients about it so that you make sure you are on target before you present the information. Your message might change depending on your audience but you always want to consider who is listening and what need you can meet.

As an example, let's say you did a special treatment for people to resolve ringing in the ears. You could find out all the challenges people have when they have ringing in their ears. Maybe they are having a hard time focusing. Maybe they can't get to sleep at night. Maybe it lowers their self esteem. You will know what these are by working with people with this problem and you can ask them about it too to learn more. Then when you are promoting your services, you can speak to these concerns. Even if people have ringing in their ears and are having a hard time focusing, they may tune into hearing you as soon as you start addressing their biggest concerns. And you can imagine, being exposed to a possible solution, there is a good chance they will seek out your special treatment. Not only because you can resolve their issue but because they can tell that you care about them since you addressed their 'pain'.

A huge reason to educate the public is that to expand your market and create more demand, you need more and more people to experience your service or product. If you only rely on the people who already are familiar with what you do to be your clients, it's going to limit you. There are millions of people who have never had a massage or facial before. There are millions of people who have never tried reflexology or a body wrap. If they don't understand what those services will do for them, they have no reason to seek them out. You need to speak to their pain and why they would want that service. I know I keep hitting on this topic, but that is why it's so helpful to have a niche because you can even be more specific on meeting their unique need or problem. You can also be strategic in what places you share this information to reach your target market.

If you are on the radio or interviewed for an article, you will be able to focus in on your expertise which makes a much more interesting conversation than something broad. You could even write an article like this yourself and feed it to a magazine or newspaper that hits your target market. I had a friend in college who was interested in journalism and so I had her conduct an interview with me and write up an article for me that I was able to use online to educate about my niche. These days, you could even create your own radio show or podcast. You could have the recording of this on your website and it's an excellent resource for people wanting to learn more about what you offer.

One way I have done recorded infomercials is through freeconferencecall.com. You can get a free phone number that you can call into and then you can record the call. Immediately after the recording, you are sent the link to the .mp3 and you can post this on facebook, a blog, your website, etc. There are many ways you could use this resource to educate the public and your customers. One idea would be to interview some of your clients who have had success with your services or products. Let their story educate the listeners and potential customers. You could also host regular conference calls where people can call in and listen or participate by asking questions. Don't be discouraged if you start this and nobody or very few people show up. If you are consistent with this over time, it will draw in more of an audience and since the calls are recorded, it gives you tons of content to add to your website. When I first started doing this I wouldn't invite anyone on. I would just record myself talking. As I gained more confidence, I opened it up for listeners to call into the line but I put them on mute. Then as I gained even more confidence, I opened it up for questions and comments. The same goes for Google Hangouts. If you are nervous like myself, take baby steps. Push your comfort zone little by little to work up to your end goal. It was also a way for me to practise before going live. As I have been doing more recorded calls and youtubes and Google Hangouts live, I am gaining more confidence. I'm sure you will find the same thing. Don't let the fear stop you from getting your message out there. You have something to offer that will help many people, but oftentimes, they need to learn about it and understand it before they pay you for it. You only get financially wealthy by people giving you money and the only way they give you money is if they believe you can meet their need or heal their pain.

When you are in a specialized field, there will be more to it than anyone really knows. You will find that people will have a lot more questions when you start talking about a very unique service or product. Educating is where you can shed light on your unique services and products. And when you are the expert, you will find that you have a lot of information to share.

Establishing yourself as the expert in your niche, will bring more opportunity to be invited onto radio shows or talk shows to educate the public about your particular area of expertise. When you are a jack of all trades but master of none, there will be less reason for someone to have you on a show. When you are the specialist in a specific field or specific service, you will be the one they will call. You could even solicit for this type of exposure by contacting talk shows or radio shows that have listeners in your target market. Radio is an excellent way to educate the public about a service or product that you offer that they may not be aware of or have little knowledge about. One reason is because they can listen to the radio while doing something else, like driving or fixing their hair in the morning. They don't have to seek out the information. A great benefit to having a niche is that the listeners are much more likely to find you after hearing you on the radio compared to if you were talking about a generic product or service that they can find at multiple salons and spas. When you are talking about a specific thing that can be hard to find and it meets their specific need, they will seek you out.

When educating the public about my niche, I would start by addressing a more general topic such as pubic hair maintenance. It is something that nearly every adult has questions about. It's not usually something a parent took time to teach their child, like other steps to proper hygiene such as brushing teeth, shaving the face, shampooing hair, etc. Many people may be curious what their options are or what is expected by their sexual partner. For a more general audience, I wouldn't start talking about all the bikini shape options or anal bleaching. I would talk about the options for pubic hair maintenance: trimming, shaving, waxing, sugaring, laser. I would address the nervousness that most people feel going to someone and showing their private parts. One of the reasons I opened Acomoclitic was because of the trouble men found finding a place to do Brazilians for men. When I first opened my shop, there were not many places that offered male Brazilians and the men that found me had often called quite a few salons before finding me. Sometimes even their inquiry about the service would be responded to as if they were asking for a sexual service and they were not treated kindly. By having a place like Acomoclitic that specialized in the service, gave new clients the comfort to call and schedule an appointment. I made it easy for people because if they called to schedule an appointment, they were most likely calling to book a Brazilian, so if all they said was that they wanted to schedule an appointment but didn't say what it was for, I didn't ask them to say out loud what it was for in case they were in a public place or even with their family and didn't want to be heard saying 'Brazilian' or 'Bikini wax'. If they called a salon that offered a lot of different services, they would have to announce what they were calling about, whereas Acomoclitic customers appreciated that they didn't need to. Our online booking was an option for added privacy. If someone wanted to book an appointment while at work but didn't want to have their entire office knowing they were booking a Brazilian, they could easily do it online. When I would be doing short talks or promos to the general public, I would focus more on these concerns because those were more likely their biggest fears regarding trying out a new service like this. I would address the benefits to having a Brazilian as it relates to hygiene. I would also suggest that it is a delicate service and to find someone like myself who specializes in Brazilians. By addressing these common concerns in my talk or interview, I was more likely to gain a new client or referral. Once they were a client, I could then discuss with them bikini shapes and anal bleaching, and educate them further on my unique niche products and services.

When educating clients one on one, I have found that it worked best to gather information about them before rattling on about my service or product. Unless their desire for your services is simply for prestige, they don't really care if the ingredient comes from some incredibly advanced process and is only available from one country in the world. They don't care if your machine is $100,000. What they want to know is how you can meet their need. You are only going to know this by asking them. Once you gather some information about their pain, then you can educate them on why your service or product is what you would recommend. You could also mention a couple things that give you credibility so they know they can trust you, but you don't need to give them your entire resume.

Educating clients one on one is where I excelled at gaining sales and you can too. In fact, when I was doing a laser consultation, I always asked the patient about their reasons for wanting the service done. This was my way of basically having them sell themselves on having the service. I would reiterate the information they gave me. If they told me it was because they were embarrassed about their hair, I would use that reason to sell them on the laser. I would get them to describe their embarrassment and how it was impacting their life. That way I could emphasize the benefits that laser would have in that particular area of concern for them. If they told me it was because shaving caused them razor burn and it was painful, I would let them know that laser would be a solution. I would ask them what their life would be like if they never had razor burn again so that they could start imaging the final results to give them a stronger desire to do the service. If they said they wanted to save money on monthly waxings or razors, I would encourage them with how much money they will save by doing the laser and even take the time to do the calculations with them so they had an exact dollar amount. Once I knew their pain, I could address it specifically instead of guessing or assuming what their specific pain was.

Since you won't have time to go into all of the benefits to laser hair removal (or whatever your service is) in a consultation, you can focus on the benefits that are most appropriate to your client. Plus if you did schedule an hour consultation so you could tell them all about laser hair removal with a power point presentation, you may be met with glossy eyes. People tune out pretty easily. In fact, during a consultation, the patient should be talking most of the time. Asking them a ton of questions and allowing them to talk about themselves will be more effective than you telling them all about yourself. After you have interviewed them, you can customize the service to meet their need. And even if it is exactly the same process as you would do to someone else, they will feel like you are customizing it for them, because they had a chance to tell you what their concerns were.

Doing presentations is another great way to educate. Once I was asked to speak, as well as demo a waxing at a leads group meeting. I'm sure this was one of the most memorable meetings they had. After I spoke about my niche and handed out brochures, I waxed a man's chest who had never been waxed before. Even though I was doing everything I could to keep the level of pain to a minimum, he still put on quite a show. When you can bring some fun and excitement into your presentations, it is much more memorable. Plus if they ever need your services, who do you think they are going to think of to call?

Another easy way to educate the public is through print, like flyers or brochures. Because there are printing costs involved, you want to be strategic in where you hand out or leave these pamphlets so you will reach your target market. They will cost time in coming up with the content, designing them, printing them and then placing them where they will be most effective. You don't want them to end up sitting in your office in a corner collecting dust. One thing I like to include are Frequently Asked Questions or Q&As. Most people have the same questions which you will find when speaking to people about your services. You can easily address these in a little pamphlet which is a great way to educate people. You can even use this pamphlet on your website. Have you ever searched for something online and you get a link to a PDF document that has the answer to your questions? That tells you that Google likes PDFs and will rank them rather high in searches. Especially when your brochure is addressing the most frequently asked questions it has a good chance of showing up in search results.

You could elaborate on the same content in a blog article or simply copy and paste the pamphlet or flyer, pictures and all right into your blog. Blogging on your website will also help you show up higher in searches and not only that, it becomes a great resource for people wanting to know more about your niche. Your website will become a great educational tool. Don't feel like you have to have everything on your website from the get go. In fact, Google likes fresh content, so adding a bit of new information every few days or weeks will be better than adding everything all at once and then leaving it.

Recently I added a chat feature on my websites and I have been getting quite a few questions coming in on a regular basis. I am having my assistant take those questions and post them on a forum in order to get the forum up and going. It's great because I'm allowing my customers to come up with half of the content which saves some energy in trying to think of those questions. Plus the forum will be directly answering people's questions, some which are commonly asked and some that could be unique.

Overtime you will become better and better at educating the public because you learn from experience. You find out what people really want to know. You find out what is the most helpful information to share. You also become more comfortable talking about your niche and you gain confidence in being the expert and having people turn to you for advice and answers. Don't feel like you have to do all of these ideas I mentioned at once. Start with one thing. Overtime, your resources for the public will grow and you will gain more exposure for new clients. I hope that you can visualize the impact that you can have by educating about your niche and how it will promote your business and draw in new clients.

Chapter 6: Add on Services

No matter which niche you choose, you still want to offer upgrades and add on services. Some of these you may not even know exist right now because you haven't yet established what your niche is. For example, before I narrowed down to Brazilians, I had never heard of anal bleaching or vadazzle. These were two add on services that I found out about as I dug in deeper to my specialty. For me, these ended up being excellent add on services because they also involved the client purchasing a product. When researching my niche, I learned that salons charged additional fees for hair buzzing prior to waxing and ingrown hair removal after waxing. I recently added butt zit cream as a product and this would be a simple treatment to add to a Brazilian too simply by applying the cream to any butt zits the client had.

On my menu of services I offered a butt facial which I called the Cheek Glow. During a Cheek Glow I would use Witch Hazel to clean the skin. Then a microdermabrasion to lift off a lot of the dead skin. Then do a mild alpha (glycolic) peel. If there were butt pimples (which was usually the reason someone was having the service performed), I would spot treat the pimples with a beta (salicylic) peel. After the peel treatment, I would do a mud mask. This was a specialty add on service I never would have thought about offering before narrowing in on my niche of Brazilians. It was an easy upsell to people with butt zits. Because it did take additional time on the schedule, sometimes I couldn't offer it the same day of the service, but could educate the client about the service and ask them if they wanted to schedule it later that week or with their next Brazilian appointment.

My friend who specialized in Brazilians offered a Vagina facial. She would include a microdermabrasion and it was something she could add onto a Brazilian that would only take an additional 10 minutes. The main reason clients wanted the service was to address ingrown hairs and you could also address things like fading dark vaginal skin, or skin tightening and firming.

A basic add on that I could easily do with hair removal, was additional body areas. The client would book an appointment for a Brazilian, but I could easily add on a brow, lip or underarm. In fact, that was one reason I didn't book myself too tightly. I gave myself room in the schedule so that I had additional time. Before leaving the treatment room, I would always ask, "Was there any other areas you wanted sugared today?" I was pleasantly surprised that more often than not, the client would say yes. If they were new clients, sometimes they even were surprised and asked "You do more than just Brazilians?" I had created such a niche for myself, they didn't always know I offered full body hair removal. Occasionally by adding on the extra areas, it would make me late for my next appointment but for the additional $25 (or whatever it was) it was worth having the next customer wait.

I can give you many ideas for add on services in my chosen niche, but what you are probably most interested in is why offering add on services is a good idea.

Some reasons for offering add ons to your niche:
-it makes you even more unique and specialized
-it adds more income, oftentimes without much more time since the client is already there
-it's a way to improve the experience for the customer
-it's a way to enhance the customer's results
-it's easy to sell
-you can gain more revenue from your customer base without expensive advertising

Add on services are a must. Like I stated before, you don't need to know exactly what they are right at this moment, but definitely be open to discovering them. And plan on having them as part of your menu. The more unique it is, the more likely someone searching online could find you...just because of your add on. Pretty cool!

Add on services don't have to be as outrageous as anal bleaching. If you are specializing in brow shaping, an add-on could be a brow tint. If you specialize in massage therapy for fibromyalgia, an add on could be hot stones or a deep muscle rub cream.

It's a great idea to have a few add on options that you can easily fit into the same amount of time allotted for the service in case you have back to back scheduled clients and can't offer upgrades that require more time. This would be things like aromatherapy, energy work, reflexology, an upgraded facial mask, a special treatment for circles under the eyes, a special lip treatment to plump or smooth the lip skin, scalp massage with a special oil, hot pack, and the list goes on. Be creative and think outside the box. You can always try out an upgrade idea for one to three months to see how clients respond and if it's something they are willing to pay extra for. By having it in a limited time frame, the clients may be more likely to purchase it too. Calculate the costs and charge accordingly so you are making a profit. Make sure the additional service doesn't put you behind schedule.

Besides add on services that you can easily do within the same appointment time, you can also offer add on services that you can sell over the phone prior to an appointment so you can book the appropriate time slot. If brow tinting is one of your add ons, when they schedule a brow wax, you simply ask them, would you also like to schedule a brow tint? If they seem unsure of what a brow tint is (which many will) this is an opportunity to educate. Remember that they are most interested in how this service will help them, not necessarily the process and it may not be for everyone so determine if it's right for them first. If they already have dark, gorgeous brow hair, they won't need it. You could ask them 'what color are your brows?' and 'do you use an eyebrow pencil?' Once you have some information about them, you can determine if the brow tinting is a good fit. If it is, you can explain, "The brow tint is designed to enhance the results of the brow wax similar to a brow pencil, but it's actually tinting the brow hair color so it won't wash off in the shower, and it will last until your next waxing appointment. It's an additional $10 and will require about 10 minutes longer for your appointment. Do you want to add on this service?" or you may ask if they have further questions about it that you can answer. Once they are interested, they may ask about the process or the product used, especially if they have allergies or have sensitive skin. This might seem like quite a bit of effort to go through for only an extra $10 but it could potentially be way more than that. For instance, if they like the service, they may add it on every month which is an additional $120 per year. If you sold 10 clients on the same thing, it's $1,200 additional revenue per year. If you sold 100 clients on the same thing, it's an additional $12,000 per year. That is the power of upsells which usually require educating the customer about the benefits of an additional service that they were not planning on having done until you explained it to them and asked them if they wanted it. If you start doing brow tints regularly on more people, you will gain invaluable experience and may become the best brow tinter around. Plus your customers will be referring more business to you because they are getting more compliments on how their brows look. Now instead of one customer spending only $15 for a brow wax, they are spending $25 for a brow wax and tint and are a much happier and loyal customer. The dollars really start to add up, and of course this is only the beginning of success if this was your chosen niche.

I mentioned up-selling your client on the phone which you will be doing in the beginning when your business is starting out. As you get busier, you won't have time to answer the phone and book appointments. When you have someone take over the phone calls for you, it is really important that you take time to train them on upselling. You can even give them incentives for upselling. I used to give my receptionist 1% bonus on total monthly sales. If I sold $25,000 she made $250 for her monthly bonus. That way she had incentive to rebook customers and upsell customers. The easiest thing to train on is suggestive selling. Even before your receptionist knows all about the services, they could at least be trained to ask the customer if they wanted to book the additional service. It could be as simple as when people called to schedule a massage that they always ask "Would you like to add on hot stones?" Suggestive selling is the easiest place to start with making more revenues with add on services. If you aren't already doing it, you will be shocked at how much more revenue you make by implementing this simple strategy. Another idea is when someone calls to schedule a massage, instead of assuming they only want an hour long appointment, you can ask them "Would you like a 60 minute, 90 minute or two hour long massage?" You will be surprised at how many people upgrade right in that moment even though they were only planning on booking an hour. Sometimes customers feel like it's too much to ask of you to do longer than an hour. But when you offer it to them, they get the impression that it's no problem for you at all. And doesn't it make sense to gain more revenue from one customer by simply asking for an upgrade, then by doing more marketing to gain a new customer for the same amount of additional revenue. Once you have a customer, and they trust you, they are very likely to spend more money with you if you ask them or educate them about your additional products and services.

In the beginning I had one client who started out as a massage client and then turned into a photofacial, brazilian wax and 2 hour massage client. Her one monthly appointment nearly covered my office rent. She wasn't able to book in advance most of the time because she travelled quite a bit with her job. Shortly after opening Acomoclitic Studio, I was feeling like I needed consistent income and applied and was hired as an assistant manager at Fascinations. I worked nights until 2am so it gave me most of the day free to run my business, but one evening I was driving to work and my client called to see if she could come in that evening for her services. I said I couldn't because I was going to work and asked if she could come in the next day. She couldn't because of her tight schedule. After getting of the phone, I wondered if I did the right thing? Maybe I should have told Fascinations I couldn't make it in that night and took my high dollar client. In fact, looking back, that would have been the smartest decision. I will never forget that day because the amount of money I made for that entire week working at Fascinations, I could have made in 3 hours with my client. It wasn't long after that, I did put in my notice and took the leap of faith that I could create the income I needed through my business and didn't need to rely on an hourly job.

I share this story not only to show how you can turn a $50 customer into a $450 customer through up sells, but also as inspiration that if you are working a regular job right now to support your business, to have a goal that you can quit your job and take your business full time and make way more income. Giving thought and attention to add on services is going to get you there faster!

Be careful not to get too crazy with too many add on services. It's best to have a few to choose from and then always be intentional about focusing on promoting one at a time. One thing to consider is the shelf life of any products needed for add ons and the overall cost to get started. Let's say you want to offer a special lip plumping service that costs $150 to purchase the kit which includes enough product for 30 treatments. How long is the shelf life of your product? Let's say it is one year. Can you sell 30 lip plumping upsells in one year? That would be 2-3 per month. If you are offering the service to every single customer, chances are you will sell all of them in the first month or two and you will have people rebooking for it. If you are only offering it on your menu but are not talking to your clients about it prior to their appointment or during their appointment, you might not even sell out in one year's time. You might even forget you have this as a service or forget how to do them. I ran into this problem at the Day Spa so I know it happens. What I learned is that it's better to have less options and that way you can pour more energy into upselling them to your clients regularly. Plus, having upsells that relate to your niche will make them more likely to be a service you are passionate about selling and offering to your clients.

If you have a lot of customers scheduling online, see if your program has a way of automatically up-selling them since you won't have the opportunity to do the suggestive up-selling by phone. Sometimes, you can have it programmed to do a pop up that encourages an upsell, or has some options that are easily visible next to the service they are booking with an explanation on why they would benefit from those add ons.

If you are ever doing a promotion on your regular service, that is a good time to offer an add on service because the customer is getting a discount on their regular service and may not mind spending some of the money they are saving. Perhaps you offer a birthday discount for 50% off your regular priced niche service so the customer is saving $30. When they call to book their appointment, you can ask them if they are interested in adding on _____ for an additional $15. Oftentimes they will because they are still saving $15 dollars off what they normally would spend. Plus, they may want to spoil themselves even more for their birthday. Not everyone is going to say yes, but it never hurts to ask...in fact it will hurt you more not to ask. Up-selling your customers on add on services is going to make you rich...or at least richer!

You have probably already been taught either in school or at your current job, how important re-booking is. I want to encourage you to take it a step further and re-book with an add on. Customers oftentimes appreciate this because they feel like you want to spend more time with them, they feel like you really care about their needs and they will re-book with the add on. An easy example would be, if you did a facial on someone and when you go to re-book you tell them about the special promotion you are offering the following month for adding a brow wax with their facial service for only an additional $5 that usually costs $15. Would they like to book the facial with the brow wax? Some people will say no to both. Some people will say they don't need the brow wax. And some people will re-book with the promotion and you just made an extra $5. If you do that with every facial client that first month, how much more income will you make the following month? If you had 40 facial clients re-book with the brow wax that would be an additional $200, easy! Plus, how many of those clients will now re-book for a facial and brow wax the following month and pay the full $15 extra instead because they loved having their brows done? Let's say half of them do. That's an additional 20 clients times $15 equals $300 extra! That additional $300 was not very hard to make. You were already going to ask for the re-book. All you did was offer an additional service at a discount. You will be happy and your clients will be happy.

In my opinion, add on services increase your client retention. Not all clients will take advantage of the add on services, but many will and they will love you for it. Don't be afraid. Decide what ones you want to offer. Decide on what specific one you want to really focus on promoting this coming month and go for it. You are going to know your clients better than me, so choose something that many of your clients can benefit from so you can offer it to every single client that books or is booked already.

Add on services will grow your business exponentially and that is why I devoted an entire chapter to the subject. I think it does take focus to sell them though, because they are often services that your current client doesn't know about or doesn't know you offer. People are busy, and they don't always take the time to read over your menu or website. That is one important reason you have to be focused and take the time to educate them and offer them on the phone, or at their appointment, or online booking. If you have a lot of different add on services, choose one per month that you focus on. That will help you sell more.

I know some people in our industry have some fears about selling.

They don't want to be pushy. That is where you really have to believe in your services and know that they are helping people. And it may help to remember that if a customer is already in your office spending money with you, they are not someone who can't afford your services. They are there because they value the service you are offering them. If you know that you can offer more to them that will help them feel better and you don't even offer it to them, it is a lose-lose. They lose and you lose. That is why it is important to know your customer's needs so you can recommend services that are going to benefit them. It could be viewed as a selfish act not to upsell if you have a service that you know will benefit your client. I understand that they will not always feel comfortable paying the additional costs. That is a risk you are going to need to take. It will push your comfort zone. But remember as you grow your comfort zone, you grow your money zone.

Chapter 7: Products that Relate to Your Niche

Once you have a niche service, it's going to be fun to learn about products that relate to that, or even create new products. Let's go back to the example of Relief-ology, Reflexology for Allergies. Imagine all of the possibilities for products that can relate to relieving allergies. What about products that can help alleviate the symptoms that people generally have from allergies? Some people get a stuffed up nose, so you could sell something like a homemade Vicks Vapor-rub. I just did a quick google search to find a recipe and there are quite a lot of options out there to give you some ideas to start with and then narrow it down to something you can make to sell with your own brand name, or maybe there's one out there that you can private label or purchase at wholesale. Another common allergic reaction are red, itchy rashes. You could sell a cream, balm or spray that would help reduce the inflammation or stop the itchy feeling, or even help with the dryness in the skin.

As you can see, once you have a niche, it is so much easier to come up with some products that would be easy for you to sell to your target market. Without having a niche, you are going to be either trying to sell everything, like a lot of estheticians, or nothing, like a lot of massage therapists. Once you narrow down your niche, you can narrow down what type of products you want to promote to your customers.

Having less products in your display case, will actually increase sales. This was a lesson learned one day after I had listened to a TED talk about merchandising. The speaker demonstrated how the research had shown that there were more purchases when there are less choices for the customer to make. I went into Acomoclitic Studio that day and took out most of the products in our display case and put them on a shelf in the back to store them. We could still access them to sell to customers on a one-on-one basis but they wouldn't be out on the product shelf as distractions. One of the products I chose to leave in the display case was our most expensive serum priced at $135. Within 3 hours of making this change, we had a customer looking at the products and asked about a couple of them and decided to purchase the expensive serum! Wow! That was fast confirmation that the speaker on TED talks knew what she was talking about. That specific serum had been on our product shelf for over 3 months and had not sold. It was too cluttered and hidden amongst all the other items. How could anyone even see it in there?

I give this example because people who listen to my advice on finding a niche service, will also want to limit their product offerings. At least the ones that are displayed in your brochure, or at the front desk, on your website, in your marketing, and of course on the product shelf in your waiting area. If you are only trying to sell a few products that relate to your unique services, they will practically sell themselves. They will be something that your target market is seeking to purchase or open to trying. However, you don't want to rely on this. It's also important to educate your clients about the products because they may have never heard of them before, and by learning more about the products and their benefits, they are more likely to purchase them. And then hopefully, repurchase them again and again. And refer others to purchase them from you as well.

If you want to earn six figures without working your butt off, you need to sell products. This is a way to make money without a ton of your time. You want your products to be unique to your brand. You want to choose products that enhance your unique niche services. These products can be bought wholesale and sold retail, they can be private label products that someone else makes but you put your brand on them, or they can be your own products that either you make or you hire a chemist to make for you.

An example of this is my friend who owns a tanning salon. She worked with a chemist to create her own unique spray tan solution. She sells small spray cans to her customers to touch up their tan in between tans. She also sells her product to other salons to use. She is currently franchising her company and then all her franchises will buy the product from her.

For My Pink Wink Cream, I purchase the cream from a chemist who makes the product for me. Then I do the bottling and labeling myself. My Gold Sugar is a product I cook myself. At Acomoclitic, one of our top sellers was a product to help reduce ingrown hairs. I am interested in making my own ingrown hair solution, but have not done that yet. I also would like to make and sell my own tweezers.

One thing I have found happening with My Pink Wink Cream and the Sugaring is that many people were buying them without ever trying out our services. They were just buying our product. Since I started selling the cream online as well as Amazon and Ebay, we have people from all over the world purchasing our product.

Products are going to be your golden ticket to making six figures or more. They are also going to support you in carving out your brand and your niche in the industry.

Since the time when I started writing this book, I sold Acomoclitic Studio but I kept my product businesses. Now I'm putting all my energy into selling products. Along with that, I started selling Nerium which is a relationship marketing product line, which is another type of way to sell products within your niche. I hadn't even thought of this before, but I am finding that for estheticians and massage therapists, it might make a lot of sense because there is low startup cost and it allows you unlimited potential as far as income. I have known massage therapists who were successful selling essential oils through network marketing. Massage therapists and estheticians would be great at marketing health products or supplements through network marketing because some of those products help with skin, acne, muscle pain, inflammation and helping people feel better. They could pick a company that has products that fit with their niche.

Whatever you choose, it helps to find something that relates to what you already do. I had tried selling discount travel through network marketing since I figured a lot of people get hair removed for vacations and it seemed like a good fit, but I had a big party and invited all of my customers. I had about 30 people come and introduced them to the company and not one signed up. Right away, it proved that my target market wasn't really into discounts on travel. It wasn't too long after that, I decided to stop selling discount travel since it was more of a distraction from my business than a helpful fit. To make things easier on yourself, if you are interested in building a product business through relationship marketing, find a product or product line that really fits with what you are already doing. For me, Nerium is a perfect fit because My Pink Wink customers and My Gold Sugar customers are already looking for ways to make their skin look better and smoother and overall more attractive. It also fits with my business of helping other estheticians and massage therapists have their own business and get rich and ultimately financially free. Make sure whatever you decide, it feels good to you and fits with your niche.

I do believe strongly that every esthetician and massage therapist as a business owner needs to include product sales as part of their business plan so they don't work their fingers to the bone. In the beginning though, you may be so focused on getting people in the door for services, products go to the way side. That is how it was for me. In fact, I shouldn't have even filed for my sales tax license my first year because once I had my sales tax license, I was suppose to report my product sales numbers monthly based on my estimated earnings which I had over estimated when applying for my license. Since I wasn't selling much (if any) products my first year, I didn't even think about filing until I was told by my accountant that I was suppose to file regardless if I had sales or not and since I didn't file, I owed money in penalties. Learn from me and don't get your sales tax license until you are making product sales regularly. In my opinion it's not worth the hassle to file until you are selling at least $100 per month or so in products. There are certain product lines that you need to provide a sales tax license for in order to buy from them, so you may need to get one sooner than later. A helpful tip would be to underestimate your earnings on the form so that you are only required to file annually, at least in the first year. You can always change it as your sales increase because you will get penalized if you are making a lot of sales and not paying taxes in a timely manner. Check with your city and state to see what their requirements are. Make a note on your calendar to file on time so you don't pay penalties. I now file quarterly but I have enough volume in sales to make it worth my time. Another thing I didn't know for a few years into business was that besides getting a Sales Tax License from the State, I also was supposed to get a license from the City. Check into this for your state and city. In Lakewood and Colorado, I am able to file and pay my sales tax online which is more convenient than mailing it in. I used to have my accountant file for me and then realized I was paying more for their service than I was in tax, so I learned how to do it myself and since it is not very difficult, I would encourage you to learn how to do it as well. If you try it a few times and decide you would rather pay your accountant to do it for you, then that will be your decision, but at least learn how to do it because it could save you hundreds of dollars.

If you use a scheduling software system that allows you to collect credit cards and payment from your customer, it might also have the option to set up the correct sales tax amount so that it calculates the correct amount for you and you remember to charge the customer. When I first opened Acomoclitic Studio, I was not using a program and I wasn't charging sales tax on the products, but when I filed my taxes, I was paying the sales tax, so basically my customers were getting an 8% discount. Once I had a software system, it made it so much easier because as soon as we added in the product to their order, the system calculated the correct amount of sales tax to collect.

Speaking of these types of systems, I do recommend getting started with one sooner than later. A couple to check out that I am familiar with are Vagaro, Booker, and MindBodyOnline. I liked having a system that I could use for scheduling, point of sale (POS), customer relationship management (CRM), emails, tweets, polls, promotions, reporting, accounting, and an online store. It made it so much easier to have everything all together, even if there were a few quirks I didn't like, I was amazed at how much these programs can do for such a small monthly cost. The sooner you get started using a program like this, the easier it will be in the long run because you will have all your clients records in one place. I also recommend sticking with one program and not jumping to a new one that comes out offering more for a better price. Chances are the one you are with will catch up to the competition with upgrades and improvements. Everytime you move to a new system, there is so much to learn and you lose a lot of information on past history. Work with what you have and learn how to utilize it to it's capacity. There are often many features included that you aren't taking advantage of. By having a system like this in place, it will also make it easy to pull the reports you need to file your Sales Tax promptly. The report will give you the exact amount of total revenue and product revenue that you need to include when filing your sales tax for city and state. You don't have to pay any federal sales tax on product sales.

There are some product lines (as you may already know) that require a minimum order to start an account with them. Before you jump into this, be certain that you have the customer base to sell the product to in a reasonable amount of time, such as three months. You don't want product sitting on your shelf for much longer than that. When you feel that you are ready to make the investment and have the customer base to support it, only order 2-3 products that you want to focus on. If you purchase the entire product line, you are guaranteed to have products sitting on your shelf collecting dust. If I was purchasing for the Golfers, I would order Sunblock, an Anti-Aging Moisturizer and some type of healing cream for sunburns with aloe vera. Those are three products that I could easily sell to every client. Plus, most golfers are men and they don't usually want to bother with special cleansers and toners. If you had a client who wanted additional products, have them pre-pay and place a special order for them to pick up.

As your business grows, you will have more money to invest in your retail products. I simply discourage you to get too over your head in the beginning when you need more cashflow to pay for rent, your backbar and daily expenses. Even putting the purchase on a credit card is not always a great idea because you can end up paying interest for months which cuts into your profits. Use caution. There were times at the Day Spa when we were re-organizing our product shelves, we would find expired products and they would end up in the trash. That was money down the drain. I have learned a lot since those days.

Even though I am focusing in this chapter on retail products, I do want to take a minute to caution against buying too much product for the back bar as well. The same thing can happen. The product sits there and doesn't get used, and if it expires you end up throwing it away and losing money. When you are starting out, don't order the big back bar sizes. Once you are busy with a full schedule of clients day in and day out, then it makes more sense to have the larger sizes. But in the beginning, a normal retail sized bottle of cleanser will last a long time. You may pay a bit more per ounce, but I still recommend it because it's less cost up front. Another suggestion that I give credit to one of my mentors Kathleen for, is to only have minimal products on your back bar. Let's say the product line you use has different cleansers, toners and moisturizers for each skin type so you want to order all the various ones for your backbar to customize your facials. Her suggestion was to only have one cleanser, one scrub, one toner and one moisturizer on the backbar. When she would recommend products for at home, then she would customize what would be appropriate for them. Not only does it save you money, it also has your treatment room looking much less cluttered. I made the mistake of ordering every single product for my backbar and it was way too much. When the lights were low, it was hard for me to see what was what, many of the products did not get used often, and it didn't make enough difference in the customer experience to justify the cost. I was thankful to Kathleen for telling me one of her secrets so I was more careful in the future to not have too many items on my back bar. Even when it came to waxing. I used the same product to prep the skin as I did to tone and soothe the skin afterwards. That saved me one less product.

For spas and salons that don't have a niche, they often have entire product lines, sometimes two or three on their shelves. Think of all the training they need to do for each new employee they hire. That is a lot of products to learn about. They would probably have higher product sales if they only sold one product line and only chose the most popular products to have on their shelf. It would be much easier to train the staff on those products and then the staff would be focused on selling those few items to their clients.

When you have a niche business, you might find that private labeling works best for your company. Since you are specializing in a specific area of concern, it seems appropriate to have your own special products. If you can hone in on 1-3 unique products that you believe in and know will help your client base, they will be easy to sell. I'm not sure what the regulations are with selling private label products online and it might depend on the company you buy from, but you may be able to open up your marketplace to include online sales.

When I first started out selling online, I was only selling from my website. Now, I sell on Amazon, eBay, Etsy, Storenvy, Openbazaar, and two of my own websites, vadazzle.com and mypinkwink.com. If you use a scheduling software that has online booking, oftentimes, they will also include an online store. This is an easy way to set up promoting your product online. I would recommend setting up links from your drop down menu to direct customers to these specific links. You can also create a page on your website describing the product benefits and then include the link to the online store to purchase the product. If you rely on the customers finding the product for sale in your software program, you won't get many sales, if any. You really need to promote the online store in other places on your website, blog, social media, youtube, and pretty much wherever you are marketing online. If you buy a domain for that specific product, let's say it's 'Hole in One Hand Cream' you can buy the domain holeinonehandcream.com and then forward the domain to the specific link on your store, or perhaps on the webpage that explains the product in detail and then has the link to the store. By doing this, you have an easier domain to use to promote your product compared to booker.com/onlinestore/holeinonehandcream12985. Does that make sense? The reason I suggest this is because having your own online store built can be expensive. If you can utilize your software program until sales support the cost of building a new online store, it saves you less up front costs. The last thing you want to do is spend a ton of money investing in an online store and getting very few sales or none at all. Once you have gained interest in the product and re-orders, then think about having your own online store. Don't be discouraged if sales are small at first. When I first started selling My Pink Wink Cream online, I was only getting a couple sales a month, then it turned into a couple per week, then a couple per day. It took years to build up to that kind of volume. Stay consistent and it will pay off. Once I listed My Pink Wink Cream on Amazon, sales really exploded.

If you list a private label product on Amazon, you need to have a barcode. You can order barcodes online. They are not very expensive. You can also use Fulfillment by Amazon (FBA) to save you time and energy filling each individual order. You basically pack up a bunch of your product and ship it to the Amazon warehouse. Then they will handle the individual orders that come in and notify you when inventory starts to get low and they need more product. They do charge extra for the service, but it allows Prime customers free two day shipping and it ends up saving you time, so I think it's worth it once you are selling product daily.

Resources I was not aware of in the beginning are programs to print shipping labels from your office so you don't need to wait in line at the post office to ship out packages. I wish I had known about this years earlier. I used stamps.com in the beginning and they have a feature that allows you to sync your eBay and Amazon orders which saves time too. Now we use ShippingEasy.com which is even nicer. They have some additional features that we like and it's all online so you don't need to download the program like we had to with stamps.com which limited us to only using one computer. Now I can print labels at home or the office. There is a monthly fee to use the service but it's totally worth it because you don't need to go to the post office. I also like having all of the information on the customers and the tracking numbers in one place so I can easily look up anything I need to compared to when I used the post office; it was easy to lose track of that type of information on the orders.

If you decide to sell products from a network marketing company, like Nerium, they handle all of the orders and shipping which is a wonderful service. I wish I would have known about Nerium years earlier at Acomoclitic Studio, because it would have been a perfect product line to sell to my customers. They offer auto-ship programs that save customers money and keep them consistent. How often have you sold a product to a customer and they never buy it again. With the auto-ship program, your customer will keep getting their product delivered until they cancel. Amazon is now offering auto-ship as well and perhaps your online store can offer it?

If you sell a professional product line, you may be restricted to selling it online. If that is the case, you may have more motivation to private label or create your own products. You can see that the online market is much wider than your local market. This would be something you could decide while putting together your business plan and long term goal setting.

I want to plant the idea that your product could be your retirement plan, whether you grow a network marketing business or create your own product(s). Selling products does not require trading time for dollars. Many estheticians and massage therapists are frustrated, especially as they are getting older, that their business cannot support their retirement. Even if they sold their business and re-invested the money, it would not be enough to sustain their lifestyle to retire. Keep in mind the option that I used, where I sold my service business but kept my product brands so I can continue to grow them and have income coming in. Whatever you decide when it comes to product sales, I suggest putting some thought into what makes the most sense for you, your clients, your business and long term plans.

Chapter 8: Teaching: Educating Your Industry

Have you noticed that many of the people who make it big in our industry end up as instructors in some way? Sometimes it's the people they have trained that may do the most instructing, but their ideas and techniques keep getting passed on and on. They become well known and can use that reputation to further their income potential. Some create their own products or systemized trainings, both of which can bring in additional revenue streams. This is when your income potential can really explode because your audience goes from your town or city where your salon or spa is, to the entire USA, or even into other countries. Without a niche to start with, it will be less likely for this to happen.

Establishing yourself as the expert in a specific service will open doors for you to start teaching classes to other professionals in your industry. Sometimes people are afraid to give away their secrets and so they choose not to teach. However, my philosophy is that I will get paid in direct proportion to the value I offer the world. With that philosophy you can never give too much.

Oftentimes, what I have found is that the people taking my classes are interested in learning 'everything.' They may never even use what I teach them, or if they do, they may use it very little in their spa or salon. There will be a few people who use it often and then there may even be a couple people who decide to specialize in it. Those couple people are not worth worrying about taking your clients. In fact, they may just happen to be your future employees, business partners or instructors!

When I first began teaching, it happened organically. People would call me and ask if I could teach them. I would tell them to find a model or two and we set up a time for a couple hours and I would teach them how to do a Brazilian or how to do sugaring. I would charge a couple hundred dollars for that type of one on one training. One lady I trained asked if she could buy sugar from me and was my first customer when I started selling my own brand of sugar. I only share this to show how all the dots come together and you can't always predict how it's all going to happen. Something to keep in mind, is the reason you are reading this book...find your niche! Having a niche is really going to open up so many more opportunities for you in the future. Being an esthetician or massage therapist who offers everything or simply the general things will not put you on the map. It will not set you apart so that other estheticians and massage therapists can find you to teach them your special skills. Does that make sense? If you want to learn how to do electrolysis, do you just look up any esthetician or salon to see if they can train you on it? Or do you look for the esthetician who specializes in electrolysis? Perhaps it's the only service offered on their website. That is the person you want to train you.

In fact, the man that trained my staff and I on our electrolysis machine is the famous Mr. Lorenzo Kunze, Sr. His niche has been hair removal, particularly lasers his whole life. I believe his grandfather created the first electrolysis machine for hair removal. He shared with me that he gets contacted often to train at different salons and spas across the country. He doesn't even solicit for those opportunities but because of his reputation within his niche market, his training is in high demand and people pay a lot for it. Even though he is retirement age and doesn't take every opportunity, he loves to do the trainings because lasers are his passion. You have the same potential.

After I had gained some notice within the Denver area for my niche, I was asked by a couple different schools to offer classes with them. I taught Brazilian classes and sugaring classes since those were my specialities. The school did most of the marketing to fill the class and I was paid a percentage of the student's tuition. I typically made $500-$1000 for the day depending on how many students and it was also an opportunity to sell some of my products. The other side benefit was that I was able to market my studio and more often than not would gain clients from the students and referrals from them as well. One of my students became a great friend and is now teaching sugaring classes, promoting and selling my products. Had I kept all of my secrets to myself, none of this could be possible. *I encourage everyone to teach others and improve our industry standard. Don't worry about giving something for nothing because ultimately it all comes back to you, even if you can't see how in the beginning.*

Videos are a great way to teach people about your speciality because it can reach a larger audience than a live class. And it is something that can become residual income. In 2007, I made a video on how to wax yourself which was to teach other estheticians how to wax themselves, or even people at home who dared to do it themselves. I hired a professional videographer. I also got a couple clients to give testimonials for the video. I had high hopes of selling a lot of the videos. One of my ideas was to sell my video to a large waxing company to include with their wax kits to help people know how best to use their product and hopefully create more regular customers but thus far that hasn't happened. (Although, you could do something like this with your specialty.) Instead, the DVD sales have been a small passive income trickling in. I have sold 180 DVDs so far at $30 each, that's $5400, over the course of nine years. My initial investment between the videographer and printing the DVDs was $1800, so it took some time to earn my money back but now it's all profit. It is a product that I can keep reprinting and selling. Awhile back, I discovered a website called createspace.com where they print and package the video as sales come in (so I don't need to pre-print them) and I get paid $8.77 for each one that sells. For a long time I had forgotten that I set this up. When doing my bookkeeping I didn't know where a mysterious deposit was coming from that said something like "Amazon credit" on my bank statement. Come to realize, I was selling 1-3 videos per month through createspace and was being paid month after month. It didn't seem like much but to date, I've been paid over $700 from that site and counting.

I was a little disappointed when I discovered that someone had uploaded the entire waxing video on youtube so people could watch the video for free. But as I got hundreds of people emailing and calling to find out about the products and techniques I was using, I realized, it wasn't such a bad thing...it was another way to market my products and brand, and help people discover me. So I went with the flow and created my own Youtube channel and started adding multiple videos with instruction on how I did sugaring and how I did Brazilians. The channel views is over 20 million and I have over 55,000 subscribers. It has turned out to be a wonderful way to promote my products and my company.

To reiterate, if I would have kept all of my secrets to myself, none of this would have been possible. I encourage you to teach what you know. I also encourage you to be taught. I have had employees in the past who thought they knew everything there was to know. Whenever I had a new training scheduled for the staff, they asked if they needed to come or not. Of course I had them come, but they came with the attitude of "There's nothing for me to learn. I know everything. I am the expert." When you become so great at what you do, it can be challenging to keep an open mind that maybe there's something more to learn. I believe one of the reasons I was able to be so successful in my career is because I have always kept an open mind to learning.

When I think back, there were two different wax classes that I went to that I learned a few new tips that I started incorporating right away into my waxing. For instance, one class the instructor demonstrated on how to hold the wax stick like a dagger when using hard wax so when you do the figure eight to apply it, you get a nice little ridge around the edges. Another class I went to with Lori Nestore (one of my greatest role models in the industry), while I was waxing legs on a model using her method, she came over to me and adjusted the way I was holding the client's leg and she corrected the tilt that I had on the spatula which made it work so much better and easier. I never went back to my old ways again.

I'm sure you can think back on some things that you have learned or re-learned that made a huge difference in your technique. There is a never ending amount to what we can learn. In our industry, there are always new products coming out so if nothing else, being open to learning about new products can make a difference for you as you become more and more of an expert in your field. One sugaring class completely altered my business and my life. Learning new techniques also keeps your passion alive and you don't get stagnant. That excitement and energy transfers to your clients. I noticed that after we had a product training with the staff, that we sold more of those products that month because of their renewed excitement and new knowledge about the products that they could tell their clients and result in a sale.

I have known teachers and instructors who simply enjoyed teaching but were not affluent. These instructors did not have a specialty. They were basically passing on the same type of information and instruction that was available in school. Of course, they had their own experiences with products and clients that they could pass on, but it wasn't anything that was going to make them rich. Having a niche business, is what is going to expand your income potential, especially if and when you become a teacher. You can charge higher prices for a class that isn't available everywhere or even for your personal reputation as the expert. For example, a class taught by Lori Nestore, the Wax Queen, is much more valuable and sought after than a wax class taught in school by someone who never was known as an expert waxer. Not only might you pay more for instruction from the expert, but you are likely to purchase their products or equipment. Don't you want to be at the receiving end of that someday, where you are the expert and they are purchasing from you? Maybe you are not ready to even contemplate these types of opportunities because you are still seeking your unique niche. I want to plant the seed so that somewhere in the back of your mind, you can see the full income potential. You can be open to the opportunities as they come to you. You may even be more prepared than I was because you are already aware that this has a high possibility of happening as you distinguish yourselves as someone who people would seek after for personalized instruction...and trade secrets. I highly recommend to not be stingy. Yet remember that your skills and knowledge are valuable and people will often pay to have you train them so be sure to charge them.

As you begin teaching, it starts to enforce your reputation as the expert. Not only will the people in our industry start to recognize you, but even your clients will have more demand for you. If you are teaching classes, make sure that your clients know. I would make announcements in my monthly newsletter promoting my classes as well as place advertisements on my website. Not only could you gain more students for your classes, but if your clients know that you are teaching other people, then they are going to have a new respect for you as their esthetician.

Depending on what you are teaching and the demand, you may find that you can make more money teaching than you can working on clients. That is not always the case, but something to research. What if you were able to make as much in one day teaching as you were working an entire month? If you are educating by doing a powerpoint presentation type style and not doing hands on where you need tables and models and equipment, you can teach hundreds or thousands of people at a time. If there is a demand for this, or you can create a demand, you could get rich pretty fast. If you charged $50 per person for your 2 hour lecture and you fit 100 people in a room, you would make $5000 in two hours. Of course you have costs involved, but you do at your salon as well. Start dreaming and making some plans on how you can make some serious money off educating. With the internet, you can offer your two hour presentation online. If you are promoting a product that you sell, you may even decide to offer the training for free knowing that it will result in product sales which could easily exceed the amount you could make from the training.

If you are interested in teaching or lecturing, I encourage you to take some classes on public speaking. The more you can learn and practise the better you will become. Toastmasters is a famous organization that helps people go from novice to great with public speaking skills. I took a course last year called Train the Trainer which was put on by New Peaks. If you are very fearful of public speaking, I encourage you that most of the best speakers were also. It's rare that someone is not afraid at first. It's like anything else in life, it takes being willing to learn to start the journey. I found that simply by being a therapist talking to so many customers, I gained more confidence in speaking. Then when I started interviewing, hiring and training staff, I became more comfortable. When I first started teaching classes, I was nervous at first but once I got into it, since it was something I knew so well, my nervousness went away. As I have pushed myself to become a stronger instructor, I do have more nervousness because I'm trying new things and pushing my comfort zone during the lectures. I believe that the more I teach, the easier it will become. When it comes to Brazilian hair removal, I could talk for hours about that service. In fact, perhaps I will write a book about it in the future. I have learned so much about that area of the body for both men and women. When I teach classes on Brazilian hair removal, I find that I can spend the entire class talking but of course estheticians really want to do the hands on, so I don't get into as much detail as I could and get right to the hands on. They are probably going to learn more by doing it than by me talking anyway. Many of your classes, might end up being primarily hands on and you won't need to become an affluent speaker. Although, it is a great skill to have regardless, and by stretching yourself, you will become a more confident person.

I did not start teaching with any thoughts of it becoming a huge money maker. I have a lot of passion to teach and help others grow and learn. Many people in our industry have that same passion and I have met kindred spirits in that regard. We want to help our clients, but we also want to help each other. All of my teachers in massage school and esthetician school made an impact on my life. I'm sure you can relate. All of the people I have learned from after that continued to enhance my skills, including people I hired that taught me new techniques and ideas. I am so grateful and I want to pay it forward. My hope is that I have inspired you to as well.

If you are interested in learning how to hire staff and contractors to grow your business and income, read my next book coming in 2017: "Hire Before You Tire: Growing Your Private Practise Beyond You."

Excerpt from Hire Before You Tire:
"When offering services, you are limited to the amount of clients you can see per day especially when you are the only technician doing the service. Not only does time limit you, but depending on how strenuous the services you offer are, you may be limited physically to a certain number of clients per day as to not overstrain your body. You may get to a point that you would like to take some time off, go on a vacation, or lower your regular scheduled hours, but still want to maintain your income level. The best solution I have for you is to hire help. Usually you need to hire when you have absolutely no time or energy to hire, but that is a sure sign that you need to hire some help. The first place to start is administration help, even 1-2 hours per day will be extremely helpful and lessen your stress. My first assistant Nancy worked for me two hours per day Monday thru Friday and my business grew from $8,000 per month to $25,000 per month within 5 months of hiring her. The second place is to pay someone (or trade someone) to help with household duties, like a personal assistant, shopping, cooking, and cleaning. This will free up your time and energy in leaps and bounds so your business can continue to flourish. Finally, if you want to go on a long vacation and make sure your clients' needs are met, you will need to train someone to cover for you. In order for your hired technician to become an expert like you, you will need to teach them everything you know. You will need to make them the expert. I chose to go this route at Acomoclitic Studio because I wanted my free time; I wanted to travel, raise a family, homeschool, and write books."

Made in the USA
Middletown, DE
05 January 2019